Praise for *PALEO DESSE...*

"Maybe you've stopped sneaking sweets, but Jane Barthelemy's new book means not giving up dessert entirely. The high-quality, nutrient-dense ingredients in these dessert recipes will help preserve and boost energy, ensuring a truly sweet ending to every meal."

—*Taste for Life*

"*Paleo Desserts* by Jane Barthelemy shows you how to indulge your sweet tooth without sacrificing your health. With 125 recipes and gorgeous color photos, Barthelemy demonstrates how to re-create classic cakes, cookies, pies, ice cream, mousses, and chocolate confections using Paleo ingredients."

—*Portland Book Review*

"The recipes include cakes and cupcakes, muffins and breads, cookies and bars, 5-minute shakes, and sauces and fillings . . . Barthelemy follows Dr. Loren Cordain's Paleolithic diet. If you are doing the same, this is a great cookbook for you."

—*Tulsa Book Review*

"For those already on the Paleo eating program, Jane Barthelemy's *Paleo Desserts* is a welcome adjunct With recipes like Black Forest Cake and Key Lime Pie, no one need feel deprived."

—*WomanAroundTown.com*

"Barthelemy has a dessert for everyone, and if you are gluten-free or grain-free you will appreciate this collection of luscious desserts."

—*San Francisco Book Review*

"*Paleo Desserts* helps create fresh alternatives to every home chef's library of favorites."

—*Midwest Book Review*

"Essential, especially for those who want to eat healthier foods."

—*Tucson Citizen*

"Barthelemy has made gluten-free, low-carb, diabetic-friendly recipes that impress."

—*RetailMeNot.com*

Good Morning
PALEO

ALSO BY JANE BARTHELEMY

Paleo Desserts:
125 Delicious Everyday Favorites, Gluten- and Grain-Free

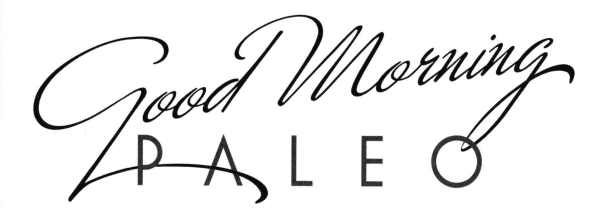

Good Morning PALEO

More Than 150 Easy Favorites
to Start Your Day, Gluten- and Grain-Free

JANE BARTHELEMY

Da Capo
LIFE
LONG

A MEMBER OF THE PERSEUS BOOKS GROUP

Library of Congress Cataloging-in-Publication Data

Barthelemy, Jane.
    Good morning Paleo : more than 150 easy
favorites to start your day, gluten- and grain-free /
Jane Barthelemy.
        pages cm
    Includes index.
    ISBN 978-0-7382-1745-1 (paperback) — ISBN
978-0-7382-1746-8 (e-book) 1. Gluten-free diet—
Recipes. 2. Wheat-free diet—Recipes. I. Title.
RM237.86.B3689 2014
641.5'63—dc23   2014001015

First Da Capo Press edition 2014
ISBN: 978-0-7382-1745-1 (paperback)
ISBN: 978-0-7382-1746-8 (e-book)

Published by Da Capo Press
A Member of the Perseus Books Group
www.dacapopress.com

Da Capo Press books are available at special
discounts for bulk purchases in the U.S. by
corporations, institutions, and other organizations.
For more information, please contact the Special
Markets Department at the Perseus Books Group,
2300 Chestnut Street, Suite 200, Philadelphia, PA
19103, or call (800) 810-4145, ext. 5000, or e-mail
special.markets@perseusbooks.com.

10 9 8 7 6 5 4 3 2 1

To my father, Richard, the creative naturalist chef,
who instilled in me a love for Nature
and a sense of wild abandon in the kitchen

CONTENTS

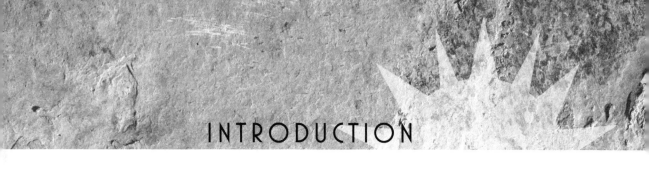

EAT BREAKFAST LIKE YOUR LIFE DEPENDS ON IT

"It's a finger snapping kind of day."
—Coco J. Ginger

Morning is the best time of day. Not that I'm a morning person—I'm definitely not. I'm a night owl. I love the morning because it holds the seeds of the day, and the possibilities are too immense to imagine. Whatever you can envision into being in the morning is what the day can become. By midmorning the day has taken on a character. And by the late night, as I try to squeeze out every last drop of experience, the day gets brittle, old, and tired. But in the early morning, anything can happen.

That's what it was like growing up with my family. My father was a wild, inspired chef, among other things, with an immense passion for food, and, yes, I'm grateful to have inherited that. He woke us up with unforgettable breakfasts and an excitement so palpable, so generous. We ate his freshly gathered wild mushrooms sautéed in butter on toast. And enormous pancakes that filled a 2-foot cast-iron pan suspended on chains over a fire in the backyard. So it was only natural for me to write this book—out of a lifelong passion for food and for the simple delight of sharing it with others.

As a child I was very robust and healthy. However, as an adult I began to be challenged with chronic fatigue, adrenal failure, allergies, and digestive problems. At one point when I was very weak and ill, I noticed there was an immediate and direct connection between what I ate for breakfast and how my day went. Of course all the meals are important, but I observed a clear response to breakfast in my body. It would accept the food with a warm feeling of happiness. Or it would shut down—a lot or a little. Call it a food reaction or an intolerance, perhaps triggered in part by an emotion. Who knows, my system would go into a tailspin—brain fog, dizziness, exhaustion, constipation, bloating, food cravings, muscle aches, moodiness, and confusion. I muddled through the day as best as I could. The only real solution was to rest and start over the next day. In time I was able to identify clearly the foods that my body accepted—fresh vegetables, tart fruits, unprocessed meats, nuts, eggs, and unrefined oils. The foods causing my body to shut down were always the same: refined carbs, grains, gluten, processed foods, milk, cheese, vegetable oils. Oh, and sugars of all kinds—even fruit sugars.

A NEW CONCEPT IN BREAKFAST

A good breakfast sets the tone for your whole day. After ten years on a diet free of grains, dairy, and sugar, my food reactions are gone. There's no morning brain fog, confusion, or any of the old discomforts. Now that I enjoy stable energy levels through the day and better health than I've had in decades, I have become a passionate Paleo enthusiast. After all, it makes sense to eat the foods we are genetically adapted to eat. That means eating

only real food. Some people might call it a limited diet. What? No bagels and cream cheese? No milk, orange juice, croissants, or Cheerios? But as you'll see on these pages, when one thinks outside the box a little bit, there is no deprivation on this diet. On the contrary—every meal is pure pleasure. My senses are clearer, my life is more enjoyable, and I accomplish more with less effort.

Our health is where the rubber meets the road. We can make the choice to listen to our bodies and harmonize with the laws of Nature. Or we can fight and suffer the consequences. Those are the two choices. This book is about using new ingredients and techniques to help you rediscover comfort foods that you thought you'd have to give up forever. So you can enjoy the pleasure of familiar flavors and textures without short-changing or undermining your health or longevity. After all, food is energy. And that energy comes from the sun. So you could say, food is concentrated sunlight. And the best foods are the highest in energetic content, the most nutrient-dense.

LICK THE SUGAR HABIT, STARTING WITH BREAKFAST

We Americans love sweets. Millions of us start the day with a donut and a cup of coffee, or perhaps a bowl of processed cereal, milk, and a banana. In many ways, we've become resigned and powerless, accepting without question an array of industrialized grains, sugar, sweets, and refined foods that are taking a huge toll on our health. After decades of daily ups and downs in blood sugar and stress levels, our bodies become established in a numbing cycle of sugar-based metabolism—call it an addiction—that eventually comes home to roost in some kind of health crisis. We lose our connection to Nature and the ability to "feel" the wisdom of our own bodies. Our current epidemic of obesity, diabetes, gluten intolerance, metabolic disorder, and a host of other maladies is linked to poor nutrition. I believe that these diseases can be prevented or healed in great part by eating a simple breakfast of real food.

The innovative recipes in this book can be a road map to a kind of metamorphosis in your life—a total change from eating processed food to eating real, original food. With these recipes you can begin to free your body of its irrational sweet cravings, and the dangerous blood sugar spikes that deplete energy and leave you wanting even more. Best of all, you can enjoy traditional breakfast favorites again, feeling deeply satisfied and nourished on every level.

WHY PALEO?

The Paleo diet, named for the Paleolithic period, mimics the hunt-and-gather food of our ancestors. Clearly they ate whatever they could catch, pluck, or dig up in the wild. During that stretch of 2.5 million years as humanity developed, our ancestors ate a diet that was fresh and alive. Fast food, industrial chemicals, processed carbs, sugars, preservatives, junk food, and even agriculture were unknown on the planet.

The Paleo lifestyle is simple and healthy. It says YES to vegetables, meat, fish, poultry, nuts, seeds, tart fruits, and unprocessed fats. It says NO to refined foods, grains, dairy, beans, extracted seed oils, and sugars. The ease of the Paleo diet is refreshing. There's no calorie counting or portion control (this part is particularly appealing). No packaged meals or special drinks. Nope, it's just a list of what to eat and what to skip. Yet the rationale behind the ancestral diet goes much deeper than physical beauty or losing weight. It's all about respecting yourself and your body, understanding your relationship to the Earth, and achieving your true human potential. Perhaps the growing appeal of Paleo is that it recalls our true primordial power and our desire to embody wholeness in a faceless industrial world.

There are many ways to interpret the Paleo diet. Obviously our ancestors ate according to the climate they lived in. Some see Paleo as a meat diet; some view it as low in carbs. Does it include eggs or fermented dairy? How about pseudo-grains like quinoa and buckwheat? These are the details, the fine print—and they're completely up to you. You can choose to emphasize meat, or you can be a Paleo-vegan. You get to decide how to interpret the ancestral diet and where you draw the line. We are all unique, and the flexible Paleo template can be molded to serve many individual needs. Since there's no counting, weighing, or portion control, the success of Paleo depends entirely on how you interpret it. This puts each of us squarely in control of our food and health.

The Paleo diet is inspired by a time when mankind ate real food. Calories don't nourish the body. Real food does. After all, food is energy, and that energy comes from the sun. Sunlight combines with nourishment from the Earth in the food we eat. We need both energy and nutrition. So a calorie as a measure of energy offers little or nothing to the body unless it is also fertile and rich in Earth nutrients from healthy soil. This is the beauty of our ecosystem in a few words. That's why 200 calories of soda will have a very different effect in the body than 200 calories of freshly picked green vegetables. When it comes to our bodies and our health, there are no shortcuts to being in balance with Nature.

The Paleo diet is a gift for millions of people with special requirements, including those intolerant to gluten and dairy, as well as diabetics and people with candida. These Paleo breakfasts can help balance the metabolism, as there's no sugar rush and subsequent energy drop later in the day. Empty calories don't exist in the Paleo world. It is a nutrient-dense diet free of the sugar and chemicals that trigger cravings and weight gain. Most people report that they lose weight on the Paleo diet and enjoy higher energy without hunger pangs or feelings of deprivation. The lifestyle also emphasizes fitness and getting plenty of sleep.

Eating healthy isn't a fad. In the final analysis, healthy eating means listening to your body and being truly sensitive to what it needs. If you've experienced health challenges, this book can be a guide to help you start anew each day. If you enjoy good health, these recipes can help you stay young and vital at any age. Every recipe is original, tested meticulously in my kitchen (sometimes up to twenty times) for flavor, texture, and body-feel.

WHAT'S A GOOD BREAKFAST?

Let's stop and think for a moment. What would you say makes a good breakfast? Well, here are my ideal requirements for breakfast:

- Tastes great
- Nutrient dense
- High in protein, moderate to low in carbs, low in sugars
- Easy to prepare
- Uses unprocessed hunt-and-gather foods
- Free of gluten, grains, dairy, sugar, beans, preservatives, industrial foods, toxins
- Compatible with your body and your diet

Surprisingly, these simple requirements eliminate most of the breakfasts we've come to accept, like cornflakes, bagels, milk, yogurt, oatmeal, and pancakes. Is it an impossible challenge? Not at all, and this book will show you how to do it step by step.

KNOW YOUR CARBS

There's a heightened awareness of carbs and sweeteners now, as processed foods are causing epidemic health challenges. Many doctors advise that a diet high in sugar and refined carbohydrates is directly linked to slower metabolism and weight gain. But how can we enjoy healthy breads, muffins, and pancakes without the "side effects," i.e., love handles that come along with them? Aha! I'll tell you the secret. To make low-carb, low-sugar breakfasts, you must use the lowest-carb flours and sweeteners. It's that simple. We're looking for ingredients that will stop the sugar cycle in its tracks.

Compare popular sweeteners and flours in the charts below. When you see the dramatic differences, you'll understand the advantages of the ingredients in this book: coconut butter, almond meal, and zero-carb sweeteners. For example, the sweetener coconut sugar is 92 percent carbs, similar to maple syrup's 89 percent. Compare that to zero-carb sweeteners Just Like Sugar, Swanson PureLo, and Swerve (See page 18 for sweetener options). If you want a low-carb muffin, which flour will you choose? Pure coconut meat and almond meal will give you a truly low-carb result, whereas tapioca flour will make your muffin high in carbs.

CARB COMPARISON IN SWEETENERS	
Sweetener	**% Net Carbs**
Just Like Sugar, chicory root	0%
Swanson PureLo Lo Han Sweetener	0%
Swerve	0%
Xylitol	72%
High-fructose corn syrup	79%
Raw honey	82%
Agave nectar	85%
Maple syrup	89%
Brown rice syrup	90%
Coconut sugar	92%
Cane and beet sugar	100%

CARB COMPARISON IN FLOURS	
Flours	**% Carbs**
Pure coconut meat	27%
Almond meal/flour	31%
Whole wheat flour	67%
Coconut flour	71%
White flour	73%
Brown rice flour	78%
Potato flour	83%
Tapioca flour	84%

A recent study by the *American Journal of Clinical Nutrition* found that foods that spike blood sugar are biologically addictive. They noticed that sugar and refined carbs cause a brain chemistry response that is a true biological addiction, lighting up the same areas of the brain as cocaine. How many of us are addicted? To find out for yourself, try eating a balanced diet that's completely free of all sugars and grains for a few days or a week. If you feel cravings, mood swings, irritability, or worse, you'll have your answer. The recipes in this book are designed to help you liberate your taste buds and your brain chemistry. They'll assist you to balance your metabolism so you are truly the master of your life.

MAKE-AHEAD, THE EASY WAY

These recipes are designed to make ahead and store, so you'll never be rushed or stumped for breakfast again—your instant meal will be waiting for you. Just a little planning is all it takes. For example, if you make a batch of twelve pumpkin muffins, freeze half of them for later. When you make a loaf of almond bread, slice it and place in a resealable bag with a piece of parchment paper between each slice. Pop it in the freezer and you'll have breakfast for several days. There are hundreds of make-ahead possibilities waiting for you.

BREAKFASTS FOR EVERY DIET

Paleo recipes are compatible with many alternative diets. You'll find an easy set of diet codes on each page. All 165 recipes are gluten- and grain-free; 164 are dairy-free. There are 79 egg-free recipes, 101 tree nut–free, 131 meat-free, and 57 vegan recipes. In addition, 162 recipes are diabetic-friendly, and 152 are candida-friendly. There are 79 high-protein recipes. And 68 recipes can be ready to eat in 10 minutes or less. For a complete chart of recipes by diet, see page 261.

RECIPES BY DIET

1. Breakfast Staples	Page	Gluten-free	Dairy-free	Egg-free	Meat-free	Tree nut–free	Vegan	Diabetic-friendly	Candida-friendly	High-protein	10 minutes or less
Coconut Butter	33	•	•	•	•	•	•	•	•		•
Homemade Coconut Milk	35	•	•	•	•	•	•	•	•		•
High-Protein Coconut Milk	35	•	•	•		•	•	•	•	•	•
Homemade Nut Milk	36	•	•	•			•	•	•		•
High-Protein Nut Milk	37	•	•	•	•		•	•	•	•	•
Flavored Coconut and Nut Milk	37	•	•	•	•		•	•	•		•
Homemade Nut Butter	38	•	•	•	•		•	•	•	•	•
Chocolate Nut Butter	39	•	•	•	•		•			•	•
Soaking and Crisping Nuts	40	•	•	•	•		•	•	•		
Homemade Bacon Bits	42	•	•	•		•			•	•	
Paleo Cream Cheese	43	•	•	•	•	•	•	•	•		•
Herbed Cream Cheese	43	•	•	•	•	•	•	•	•		•
Paleo Feta Cheese	44	•	•	•		•	•	•	•		•
Paleo Butter	45	•	•	•	•	•	•	•	•		•
Paleo Omega-3 Butter	45	•	•	•		•	•	•	•		
Perfect Coconut Pie Crust	46	•	•		•		•	•	•		
Homemade Bone Broth	47	•	•	•		•		•	•	•	
Fermented Veggies	48	•	•	•	•	•	•	•	•		

THINKING OUTSIDE THE CEREAL BOX

Eating original food in this way will bring health and peace to your body. You'll be amazed at how much better you feel through the day, at your higher energy levels, and the ease with which you drop those extra pounds. As your cravings dissolve and you feel at home in your body again, you'll experience a continual and growing freedom from old eating habits—yes, most of us would call them addictions. Giving up sugars may challenge your deepest psychological corners, and these recipes will provide a smooth, comfortable transition without deprivation. All it takes is simply walking away from the masquerade of empty industrial food, and delighting in the joys of real nourishment.

By eating real foods and reducing consumption of sugar and processed carbs, the body intelligence can finally shine through, and slowly we begin to heal from the inside out. When we harmonize our bodies and our kitchens with Nature, it's a new day and a new beginning in ways we can't even imagine. With a jump-start of a great breakfast, you'll have a firm energy foundation to step out of your past and embrace whatever your future holds.

————————

INGREDIENTS

"You are what you eat,
so don't be fast, cheap, easy, or fake."
—Anonymous

The recipes in this book use real food, as fresh as possible. In a Paleo breakfasts book, you can expect to find some rather unusual ingredients, and I've done my best to help you find them. Some of the more "interesting" ingredients are coconut butter, arrowroot flour, chia seeds, and nutritional yeast. They're all used for specific reasons of taste or texture and are necessary parts of the recipe. I suggest you follow a recipe exactly at least the first time, and after that you can vary it to your taste. You will be more successful if you wait to experiment or substitute ingredients until the second or third time you make it. These ingredients are all staples in my tiny Paleo kitchen. If I can do it, I know you can do it, too.

AÇAÍ BERRIES

The açaí palm tree native to Central and South America produces a delicious berry that is high in antioxidants. Pure açaí pulp is delightful in smoothies. Find Sambazon Smoothie Packs—Unsweetened Açaí Berry Purée in some healthy groceries or amazon.com.

AGAR POWDER

Agar is a tasteless white seaweed and a fantastic thickener from Asian cuisine that dissolves instantly in boiling water and thickens when heated much like albumen in eggs. Agar is especially useful in grain-free, egg-free muffins, such as Apple

Spice Muffins (page 145) and Lemon Chia Seed Muffins (page 149). A teaspoon of agar powder is equal in thickening power to 3 teaspoons agar flakes, which are available in most grocery stores; however the flakes are costly and require blending to dissolve. You can buy Frontier brand agar powder at amazon.com.

ALMOND MEAL

One of the best grain-free flours available, almond meal is highly nutritious, low in carbs, and available in any grocery. You can also use almond flour, which is often a finer grind, in these recipes—I use them interchangeably. However I have found that with a good leavening balance, almond meal works just as well, is economical, and is more widely available. I use almond meal in breads, pancakes, and pastries. These recipes are tested with almond meal made from blanched, skinned almonds. If you're grinding whole almonds into flour including the skins, note that this is not the same ingredient, and the amount required may be different. Find almond meal in any healthy grocery, bobsredmill.com, or nuts.com.

APPLE CIDER VINEGAR

Raw, fermented apple cider vinegar has powerful health benefits. Look for unfiltered, unpasteurized organic vinegar that contains the "mother." This is a natural sediment that you can see floating at the bottom of the bottle. Apple cider vinegar is a probiotic that aids digestion, promotes the growth of healthy microflora, restores your body's natural pH balance, and helps to control sugar cravings. Buy it in any healthy grocery or online at bragg.com.

ARROWROOT FLOUR

This is a very finely ground root powder that I use as a gluten-free binder in baked goods and even pancakes. It is an excellent substitute for cornstarch or potato starch. Since both these are common allergens, arrowroot has the distinct advantage that it is neither a grain nor a nightshade plant. Find it in any healthy grocery or at vitacost.com or bobsredmill.com.

BAKING SODA

The only Paleo-friendly leavener, sodium bicarbonate comes from a natural mineral that was originally mined. Baking soda gives great results in your baked goods. An alkaline, when mixed with an acid such as vinegar or lemon juice, it releases air bubbles to raise your muffins. Baking soda will lose its potency over time and should be replaced every three months.

BEE POLLEN

Bee pollen is the food of the young honeybees. It's a superfood for people, too, as it contains nearly all nutrients required by humans. High in protein, as well as free amino acids, vitamins including B-complex, and folic acid, I use it in smoothie recipes. Find it in any healthy grocery or at iherb.com or vitacost.com.

BUCKWHEAT

It's not a grain, nor is it related to wheat, but is instead a distant relative of rhubarb. Buckwheat makes a flavorful alternative to grain that's gluten-free and Paleo. Buckwheat is high in protein, phytochemicals, antioxidants, and fiber. Like all seeds and nuts, it is best soaked overnight. Buy raw buckwheat groats in the bulk section of healthy groceries or at bobsredmill.com or vitacost.com.

CACAO POWDER AND CACAO NIBS

I use pure cacao powder and occasionally unsweetened cacao nibs. It is important to check the ingredient label, since many chocolate products contain sugar, milk, or soy lecithin. Look for 100 percent pure cacao that's completely sugar-free. Buy pure cacao powder and cacao nibs in healthy groceries or at vitacost.com, navitasnaturals.com, or sunfood.com.

CAROB POWDER

Carob comes from the pod of a tree in the Mediterranean region. Its pulp is sweet, mild, and chocolate brown in color. Carob powder can be substituted for cacao powder one-for-one in recipes. Unlike cacao, carob contains no caffeine, an advantage for children or people with caffeine sensitivity. I use it in sweet recipes to impart a rich dark color. Find it in any healthy grocery or at vitacost.com or bobsredmill.com.

CHIA SEEDS

A highly nutritious superfood, chia seeds are high in omega-3 fatty acids. These amazing seeds expand when mixed in liquids, so they make a high-protein binder and thickener. I use both black and white chia seeds, however I prefer the white ones for light-colored breads and baked goods, to mimic the color of traditional breads. Look for black and white chia seeds in most healthy groceries. For the best prices online and in bulk, check out vitacost.com, amazon.com, chiaseedsdirect.com, healthworksllc.net, or nutsinbulk.com.

CHICORY ROOT GRANULES, ROASTED

Naturally caffeine-free chicory root granules add a rich, satisfying flavor to Cappuccino (page 98), plus they are high in antioxidants that support healthy liver function. I buy the granules in bulk online and brew with roasted dandelion root for a delicious Paleo coffee substitute. Look for Frontier brand at amazon.com.

CHLORELLA POWDER

Chlorella is a single-celled green micro-algae. When dried it is about 45 percent protein, an excellent vegan source for complete protein. Chlorella is high in antioxidants, vitamin C, and carotenoids and is considered one of the most powerful supplements to eliminate toxins. I use it in smoothies and as a superfood addition to baked goods. Find in most healthy groceries, from an herb specialist, or at sunfood .com, vitacost.com, or mountainroseherbs .com.

CHLOROXYGEN

Chlorophyll is the green pigment in plants, involved with photosynthesis, which produces oxygen. Chlorophyll concentrate helps to rebuild red blood cells and hemoglobin, restoring the blood's oxygen-carrying capacity. ChlorOxygen by Herbs Etc. increases the amount of oxygen available to cells. I use this in smoothies. Find it in any healthy grocery or at luckyvitamin .com or vitacost.com.

COCONUT AMINOS

Coconut aminos are a liquid seasoning made from pure aged coconut sap with salt. Similar to soy sauce (except it is gluten- and soy-free!), it adds flavor to savory sauces and stir-fries. Find in any healthy grocery or at iherb.com or vitacost.com.

COCONUT BUTTER

Also called coconut cream concentrate, or coconut manna, it is simply coconut meat ground into butter. Coconut butter has many advantages: It is hypoallergenic and tree nut–free; it contains one-quarter of the carbs in wheat flour or processed coconut flour; it is an unprocessed, highly nutritious whole food. And it is pure coconut meat, without any filler from the hull or husk. Homemade coconut butter is one of the most economical gluten-free flour substitutes available. It is easy to make in a super blender or food processor for a fraction of the store price—see the recipe on page 33. Use it in so many tasty breakfasts, from muffins to quick breads, pancakes, and dairy-free cheese. Luscious and rich, it is one of my favorite ingredients. Coconut butter is quite hard at room temperature; it softens at 78°F. To soften it for easy measuring and hand mixing, place the container in a bowl of warm water. There are two ways to measure coconut butter. Cold, solid coconut butter is easy to measure by weight, but more difficult to accurately measure when pressed into cups. Softened coconut butter is easy to measure in cups and is also easy to weigh. When using a food processor, you can save time by adding the cold coconut butter in chunks and let the machine grind it for you. If you're mixing by hand, you'll need to soften it first. Buy coconut butter in any healthy grocery or at artisanafoods .com or vitacost.com.

COCONUT FLOUR

I use coconut flour in a few recipes for its superior absorption qualities and for flouring pans. It has a somewhat dry, grainy texture to my palate, and it is pricy, so I do not use it much. Made from processed, defatted coconuts including the husk and hull, coconut flour is high in fiber and light brown in color, though sometimes it is bleached to make it white. Instead I prefer coconut butter as a luscious whole-food alternative—it's made from pure white coconut meat without the extra filler from the husk and hull, and it's very economical homemade. Buy coconut flour in any healthy grocery, at bobsredmill.com or vitacost.com.

COCONUT MILK

Homemade coconut milk is my go-to nondairy milk; it's perfect for smoothies, quiches, cheese sauces, and as a topping for fruit. Make it yourself in minutes for the most economical way to enjoy it. All you need is a blender (any kind will work), and you can drink it in minutes—see the recipe on page 35. I also use canned BPA-free coconut milk, full fat, as thick as possible. My favorite brand is Native Forest organic by Edward & Sons. Look for unsweetened full-fat coconut milk (not "lite") without additives or guar gum. Coconut beverages in a carton will work in some of these recipes, but I do not recommend them as most contain added water, sweeteners, and stabilizers. Buy Native Forest organic canned coconut milk in any healthy grocery or at vitacost.com or edwardandsons.com.

COCONUT OIL

Unrefined virgin coconut oil can withstand high temperatures in baking and frying and is easy to store—making it a great Paleo oil. Even better, it's widely available, and it tastes great. Coconut oil is solid at room temperature. However, it melts easily at 78°F. To soften it, place the jar in a bath of warm water. Find unrefined coconut oil in any healthy grocery or at tropicaltraditions.com, vitacost.com, or nutiva.com.

COCONUT, SHREDDED

Shredded coconut flakes are pure white grated coconut meat that is not otherwise processed. It is a tasty whole food, highly nutritious, economical, and widely available. You can grind it in a super-blender such as the Blendtec or Vitamix or a food processor to make your own homemade coconut butter (page 33) for a fraction of the store price. When shopping, you'll want to look for full-fat coconut flakes. Find it in the bulk bins in any healthy grocery or at vitacost.com or tropicaltraditions.com.

COCONUT WATER, UNSWEETENED

Coconut water is the nutritious clear liquid from inside a coconut fruit. I use it in smoothie recipes. It's high in nutrients such as lauric acid, chloride, and iron, as well as electrolytes such as potassium, magnesium, calcium, sodium, and phosphorous. The potassium content in coconut water is almost twice that contained in a banana. Find it unsweetened in any grocery store.

CRYSTALS, VITAMIN C

Vitamin C imparts a tart taste like lemon or sharp cheese in recipes. Also called ascorbic acid crystals, it is a common vitamin supplement. Look for pure vitamin C with no added ingredients. The crystals dissolve instantly in water. If you consume a lot of ascorbic acid on an empty stomach, it can cause indigestion, so go easy. Find vitamin C crystals in the supplements section of any healthy grocery or at iherb.com or vitacost.com

DANDELION ROOT GRANULES, ROASTED

Dried, roasted dandelion roots add a rich and satisfying flavor to caffeine-free Cappuccino (page 98). Dandelion is a powerful liver cleanser and digestive tonic. I buy the roasted root granules in bulk online and brew them with roasted chicory root for a wholesome, full-bodied beverage. Find them under the Frontier brand at amazon.com.

EGGS

The best eggs are from happy, healthy chickens at your local farm, where they get to roam outside most of the time, eating a diet that is GMO- and chemical-free. I also use pasture-raised organic eggs from the grocery store. Egg size can vary, and this can be critical in some recipes. When in doubt, you can weigh your eggs on a digital scale—a standard large egg is 55 grams.

FLAXSEEDS, FLAX MEAL, AND FLAX OIL

Flaxseeds are a powerful source of omega-3 fatty acids, lignans, and fiber. Remember to grind them. A hand-held grinder or super-blender such as the Vitamix or Blendtec is useful for this purpose. Preground flax spoils, or oxidizes, quickly. Unground, the seed's impermeable coating may make it pass right through your digestion, without imparting any of the benefits. However, ground flaxseeds, called flax meal, is a wonderful superfood. I use flax meal in uncooked cereals, and I use the oil in smoothies. I do not cook with flax seeds, meal, or oil, as the delicate oils can become unstable when heated and create free radicals in the body. Find whole flaxseeds in any healthy grocery or at bobsredmill.com or vitacost.com.

GREEN POWDER

Dark green powders are concentrated nutrition with vitamins, minerals, amino acids, antioxidants, phytonutrients, and chlorophyll. Made from dehydrated leafy greens, the best green powders often have a bitter flavor. Start with a small scoop and increase the dose as you get used to it. You may find you enjoy the natural bitterness as a morning tonic. Look for an unsweetened powder such as VitaMineral Green by HealthForce Nutritionals available from vitacost.com or healthforce.com. I also like Body Ecology Vitality SuperGreen Powder, available from bodyecology.com or amazon.com.

GOJI BERRIES

This bright orange-red berry from China is called a superfood because of its immune-enhancing antioxidants and vitamins. It comes from a nightshade plant related to the tomato. Find dried goji berries in most healthy groceries or at navitasnaturals.com or vitacost.com.

HEMP NUTS

A true superfood, hemp nuts contain the ideal balance of amino acids and fatty acids necessary for human health. I use them in hemp milk, hemp butter, and grain-free cereals. Hemp nuts are delicate and should always be refrigerated. Also called hemp hearts and hemp seeds, you can find them in any healthy grocery or at nutiva.com or vitacost.com.

HOLY BASIL OR TULSI TEA

Ayurvedic medicine has long used holy basil, or Tulsi, as an herb to treat stress naturally. It has a flavor similar to black tea and works as an adaptogen to help the body naturally cope with stress. I use it in Chai Tea (page 99) because it tastes wonderful and is caffeine-free. Buy Organic India tea bags in any healthy grocery or at swanson vitamins.com or iherb.com. Save money buying in bulk at starwest-botanicals.com or oregonswildharvest.com.

HONEY

Raw honey is a true Paleo food that is about one and one-half times sweeter than sugar. I adore the flavor of honey. However, it is very high in carbs and calories. Honey will give you a nice big blood sugar spike and won't help you kick the sugar habit. So it's best to use it in very small quantities and reserve it as a rare Paleo treat. Find raw honey in some healthy groceries or at honeylocator.com, swansonvitamins.com, or vitacost.com.

KEFIR

This fermented milk beverage originated in Caucasus Mountains thousands of years before refrigeration. You can make it yourself by adding kefir grains to fresh milk. It's not quite Paleo as it contains dairy; however, many dairy-intolerant people can digest it and benefit from it, especially goat kefir. Kefir is a potent probiotic and rich in vitamin K-2. You can make coconut kefir that's 100 percent dairy-free and Paleo. When buying cultured coconut milk, check the ingredients and avoid brands that contain additives and sweeteners. You can buy pure goat kefir in most healthy groceries.

MACA POWDER

Maca is a root from the high Andes Mountains. Sometimes called Peruvian Ginseng, maca is known as an adaptogen, meaning it helps to regulate metabolism, build the immune system, and increase endurance. It has an earthy, slightly sweet taste and is often paired with chocolate. Buy it in some healthy groceries or at navitasnaturals.com or vitacost.com.

MAPLE FLAVOR

I use maple flavor occasionally to recall the flavor of maple syrup. Just a little bit adds a full-bodied maple taste. Look for a GMO-free maple flavor such as those available at baktoflavors.com.

MEATS, POULTRY, AND FISH

The ancestral diet contained wild meats, fowl, and fish. In the twenty-first century, that means choosing the best quality meats that are as close as possible to the wild version. In these recipes I use wild salmon, pasture-raised chicken, bacon, ground meats, and organ meats such as liver and kidney. Look for unprocessed, sugar-free meats from grass- or pasture-raised animals that have a diet free of antibiotics, GMO grains, and chemicals. In other words, the best nutrition will be from a happy animal, raised with loving care. For local sources in the United States and Canada, see the guide at eatwild.com.

NUT MILKS

Nut milks are a snap to make, and they taste luscious. The creamy, real-food flavor is far superior to expensive, store-bought beverages, and you'll never want to go back. I use a variety of nut milks in smoothies, quiches, and sauces. You can make milk from any nut or seed, such as almond, hemp, and pumpkin. See the easy recipe on page 36. Why pay more for imported, chemical dilutions, when you can make it fresh and quicker yourself?

NUTRITIONAL YEAST

A popular vegan condiment, nutritional yeast has a nutty, cheeselike flavor. Nutritional yeast comes from a single-celled organism, *Saccharomyces cerevisiae*, which is washed and dried with heat to deactivate it. It is an excellent source of protein and vitamins, especially B-complex vitamins, and it is a complete protein. It is also free of sugar, dairy, and gluten. I use it to add a cheesy taste to sauces and eggs. Find it in healthy groceries, bragg.com, bobsredmill.com, or vitacost.com

NUTS AND SEEDS

An excellent source of protein, nuts add texture and flavor in baked goods and grain-free cereals. I use almonds, walnuts, pecans, pumpkin seeds, sesame seeds, sunflower seeds, hemp seeds, etc. Nuts contain bitter coatings that harm the digestion; however, it is easy to remove them by soaking. When nuts are soaked and lightly toasted, they are truly digestible and healthy. See Soaking and Crisping Nuts (page 40). Look for the freshest organic nuts in a healthy grocery or at sunorganicfarm.com, tierrafarm.com, rawnutsand seeds.com, or wildernessfamilynaturals.com.

OLIVE OIL

A true Paleo food, olive oil is not an extracted seed oil. It is the whole olive crushed and filtered. I use olive oil in raw and cooked dishes such as Paleo Feta Cheese (page 44), Paleo Butter (page 45), Rosemary Olive Bread (page 63), and Personal Pizza for One (page 180). It's especially wonderful in dishes that need that rich Mediterranean flavor. Stored in a cool dark place, a quality extra-virgin olive oil can withstand baking and be a healthy addition to your diet without worries of oxidation.

ONION FLAKES, DEHYDRATED

Dehydrated, chopped onions are easy to use and add a flavor boost to savory recipes. Find them in the bulk herbs section of healthy groceries, wildernessfamilynaturals.com, or frontier.com.

PALM OIL

Palm oil comes from the reddish pulp of the oil palm fruit. That's why unrefined palm oil is reddish in color; and it's loaded with natural vitamins, carotenes, and antioxidants. White palm oil is the refined version—processing removes its color, flavor, and most of the health benefits. I don't use much palm oil because of deforestation and habitat destruction associated with its production. Buy red palm oil in healthy groceries or at tropicaltraditions .com or nutiva.com.

PROTEIN POWDER

I use protein powders in smoothies and superfood recipes. There are many protein powders available. Look for an unsweetened powder without a lot of fillers. I like Bluebonnet Whey Protein Isolate, Original recipe, which is unsweetened. I also use NOW 100% Egg White Protein. Find Bluebonnet Protein Isolate, Original recipe at iherb .com. Find NOW 100% Egg White Protein at swansonvitamins.com or amazon.com.

SALT, UNPROCESSED

One-hundred-percent unprocessed salts such as Himalayan salt, Celtic salt, and unprocessed sea salt will give a delicate flavor to your recipes without any added chemicals. Find finely ground salts in any healthy grocery or at swansonvitamins .com or vitacost.com.

SEAWEED, HIZIKI, AND WAKAME

Dried seaweed has many health benefits. It is high in fiber and essential minerals such as calcium, iron, and magnesium. Use hiziki and wakame seaweeds interchangeably—they are thin strands, deep green, almost black in color. I soak them in hot water for a few minutes and add them as superfoods to baked goods. Buy seaweeds in most groceries or at vitacost.com or edenfoods.com.

SWEETENERS

Sweeteners are a favorite subject for me, and one I have researched in depth. These recipes are the synthesis of that research. This book is about delicious recipes that promote a balanced metabolism and level blood sugar all day, starting with breakfast. That's why I do not use many of the common so-called "natural" sweeteners. For more details on sweeteners, see my website GoodMorningPaleo.com.

The best Paleo sweeteners are low in sugars and carbs and won't affect blood sugar. In these recipes, the sweetener measure is based on table sugar, or Just Like Sugar Table Top natural chicory root, which are measured cup for cup the same. Other sweeteners I recommend are Swanson PureLo Lo Han Sweetener, Swerve, and raw honey. To use these, you may need to convert. Don't worry—I've mapped it all out for you in the charts on page 20.

Choose Your Sweetener

I encourage you to experiment with sweeteners to find one that works best for you. These recipes are designed to use the zero-carb sweeteners below. However, you may substitute any other sweetener, knowing that it will alter the flavor and carb profile of the finished recipe. (Note that I do not use agave, maple syrup, coconut sugar, or xylitol as they are very high in carbs and will cause blood sugar to spike. I do not use refined stevia powder or liquid, as they are highly processed with chemicals.)

Just Like Sugar Table Top is a natural chicory root sweetener that is easy to measure cup for cup like sugar. After testing hundreds of sweeteners I find it dissolves easily and tastes like table sugar. A zero-calorie, zero-carb sweetener, it does not affect blood sugar. It gently sweetens everything without the usual sugar spike and the drop soon after. There are three varieties of Just Like Sugar: Table Top, Brown, and Baking. The Table Top version gives the best flavor and texture in baked goods. Just Like Sugar Brown is similar to the Table Top version. It has the additional ingredient of concentrated steam from molasses, which is dehydrated to create a brown sugar flavor that's healthy and nonglycemic—an amazing invention! I use both Table Top and Brown. The Brown has a rather strong flavor, so I like to mix them half Table Top, and half Brown. (I do not recommend the Baking version, as it has a higher fiber content, is measured by weight, and cannot be used cup for cup like sugar.)

Just Like Sugar is made of crystal chicory root that is 96 percent dietary fiber, mixed with calcium, Vitamin C, and pure orange peel. Chicory root fiber is high in fructo-oligosaccharides, which taste sweet but do not affect blood sugar or cause weight gain. A natural probiotic, chicory root inulin helps to promote healthy intestinal flora. Powdered orange peel is a highly concentrated sweetener that is six hundred times sweeter than sugar. Let me say right away that I am not paid or endorsed by Just like Sugar in any way—I just like their sweetener. Buy Just Like Sugar, both Table Top and Brown, at vitacost.com or justlikesugar.com.

PureLo Lo Han Sweetener by Swanson is made from lo han guo, a sweet Chinese herb also called monk fruit. It is mixed with pure white inulin powder and is approximately six times sweeter than sugar. I find it has a gratifying sweet flavor and no aftertaste. Even better, it has zero carbs, zero calories, and contains no sugars. Find it online at swansonvitamins.com or amazon.com. Unlike Just Like Sugar, the ratios are not cup for cup; see the conversion chart below.

Swerve sweetener is a blend of erythritol, a fermented sweetener. It is made from non-GMO vegetables and fruits. It has zero calories and does not affect blood sugar. Erythritol works well in baked

goods. I find it does not always dissolve completely in cold dishes. It is used cup for cup like sugar. Find it at swervesweetener .com or vitacost.com.

Raw honey is a natural Paleo sweetener that is about 1½ times as sweet as sugar. It contains almost the same amount of sugar as table sugar. These recipes are all diabetic-friendly, provided that you use only the zero-carb sweeteners recommended above. Honey is not diabetic-friendly. It will give you a nice big sugar spike, so go easy. Buy raw honey in most healthy groceries or at swansonvitamins.com or vitacost.com. As with PureLo, you'll need to make a conversion for honey—see the chart on page 20.

Note: These simple sweeteners are safe and healthy for the vast majority of people, including those with gluten intolerance, celiac disease, and diabetes. However, every person's digestion is unique, therefore these products may not be suitable for everyone. For example, a few people suffering from IBS or SIBO may not tolerate chicory root fiber. Before starting any new diet, please check with your medical practitioner.

Choose Your Sweetness Level

How sweet do you like your muffins? Some people like them very sweet, and others prefer little or no sweetener. After a time on a low-sugar Paleo diet, many people notice they need less sweetener. I find there's a huge range of preferences regarding sweetness level in baked goods.

These recipes are designed to give you a medium sweetness. If you like a low level of sweetness, start with half the amount of sweetener called for in the recipe. Then taste the mixture and sweeten to your own taste. If you prefer a high sweetness level, start with the amount called for in the recipe. Then taste the batter and add more a bit at a time, to taste. Sweetener can be added at any point.

Sweeteners Recommended	Comes From	% Net Carbs	Carbs per Cup	To Replace 1 cup sugar
Just Like Sugar Table Top	Chicory root	0%	0	1 cup
Just Like Sugar Brown	Chicory root	0%	0	1 cup
Swanson PureLo Lo Han Sweetener	Lo han guo	0%	0	2½ tablespoons
Swerve*	Erythritol	0%	0	1 cup
Raw honey**	Honeybees	82%	275	⅔ cup

*Dissolves best in heated recipes.

**For every cup of honey, use ¼ cup less liquid, add ½ tsp. soda, and reduce the temperature by 25°F.

SWEETENERS—EASY CONVERSION CHARTS

RAW HONEY	
Sugar = 1	Honey = ⅔
If recipe calls for:	Use this much raw honey:
1 tablespoon	⅔ tablespoon
2 tablespoons	1⅓ tablespoons
3 tablespoons	2 tablespoons
¼ cup	2⅔ tablespoons
⅓ cup	3⅔ tablespoons
½ cup	⅓ cup
¾ cup	½ cup
1 cup	⅔ cup
1¼ cups	¾ cup
1½ cups	1 cup
1¾ cups	1 cup + 2½ tablespoons
2 cups	1⅓ cups

SWANSON PURELO LO HAN SWEETENER	
Sugar = 1	Swanson PureLo Lo Han Sweetener = ⅙
If recipe calls for:	Use this much Lo Han Pure:
1 tablespoon	½ teaspoon
2 tablespoons	1 teaspoon
3 tablespoons	1½ teaspoons
¼ cup	2 teaspoons
⅓ cup	1 tablespoon
½ cup	4 teaspoons
¾ cup	2 tablespoons
1 cup	2⅔ tablespoons
1¼ cups	3⅓ tablespoons
1½ cups	¼ cup
1¾ cups	5 tablespoons
2 cups	5⅓ tablespoons

PureLo Lo Han Sweetener by Swanson is six times sweeter than sugar.

WHAT'S *NOT* IN THESE RECIPES?

Well, frankly, a lot:

- There are no grains such as wheat, barley, rye, corn, rice, or oats.
- No beans such as soy, tofu, pinto beans, lentils, or chickpeas.
- No dairy, milk, cream, yogurt, or cheese (except for one smoothie with goat kefir).

- No sugars or refined sweeteners like maple syrup, coconut sugar, agave, stevia, and no artificial sweeteners.
- No sweet fruits such as pineapple or mango. No dried fruits such as raisins and dates.
- No extracted seed oils, such as canola, soy, corn, safflower, etc.

————

YOUR PALEO
KITCHEN-SHOPPING CHECKLIST

*"Shop on the edges of the supermarket where you'll find the fresh foods.
Avoid the processed foods in the middle."*
—Michael Pollan

An organized kitchen is a joy to work in. Here's how I set up my pantry. I keep a shopping list on the fridge and circle an item when it's needed. Before shopping, make a plan of what you'd like to eat for the next week, and make a shopping list. Use the checklist on the next page, or write your own. In the grocery store, stick to your list. Focus on fresh produce and meats. Try to shop on a full tummy, as hunger can lead to impulse shopping. Shop without children if possible—they are the ultimate impulse shoppers.

Clean Paleo shopping means avoiding certain foods. Stay out of the processed aisles if you can. Steer clear of grains, and read the labels. Avoid sugar under names like maltodextrin, cane juice, coconut sugar, molasses, agave, maple, dextrose, fructose, or anything ending in "ose." If an item has more than five ingredients or you can't pronounce them, put it back on the shelf.

In the produce section, pass up high-sugar fruits such as bananas, pineapples, and grapes. Instead, go for tart fruits like Granny Smith apples, lemons, limes, and blueberries. Look for seasonal dark green veggies like kale, spinach, chard, and beet tops, which are nutrient dense and economical.

In the meat department, ask for organic, or grass-fed, grass-finished meats without antibiotics, hormones, sugar, or GMO grains. Be wary of misleading terms such as "free-range" or "natural" that may not indicate the best quality.

For sources, see Ingredients (page 9) or Buying Guide (page 271).

SHOPPING CHECKLIST AND STORAGE GUIDE		
Refrigerator	**Pantry**	**Spices and Flavorings**
Bee pollen	Almond meal	Agar powder
Chlorella powder	Apple cider vinegar	Allspice, ground
Coconut aminos	Arrowroot flour	Almond extract
Eggs, pastured organic	Baking soda	Anise seeds, ground
Fermented veggies	Buckwheat	Bay leaves
Flax oil	Cacao powder, cacao nibs	Black pepper
Flax seeds, whole	Carob powder	Caraway seeds
Fruits	Chia seeds, black and white	Cardamom, ground
Goat kefir	Chicory root granules, roasted	Cayenne powder
Green powder	Coconut butter	Chile molido or chile powder
Hemp nuts	Coconut flour	Chipotle powder
Kalamata olives	Coconut milk, canned	ChlorOxygen
Meats	Coconut oil	Cinnamon, ground
Nut butters	Coconut, shredded unsweetened full-fat	Cloves, ground
Nut milks	Coconut water, unsweetened	Coconut aminos
Nuts and seeds	Dandelion root granules, roasted	Crystals, vitamin C
Vegetables	Green chiles 7-oz. can	Cumin, ground
	Hiziki or wakame seaweed	Decaffeinated coffee crystals
Freezer	Holy basil or Tulsi tea	Fennel seeds
Açaí berries, Sambazon Smoothie Packs, unsweetened	Honey, raw local	Ginger, ground
	Just Like Sugar Brown	Maple flavor
Prepped breakfasts	Just Like Sugar Table Top	Nutritional yeast
Cubes of jams, ketchup	Maca powder	Onion flakes
Cubes of bone broth, pâté	Olive oil	Paprika or smoked paprika
Paleo cream cheese	Parchment paper	Pumpkin pie spice
Paleo feta cheese	Protein powder	Rosemary leaves
	PureLo Lo Han sweetener	Sage powder
	Red palm oil	Salt, unprocessed
	Sesame oil, toasted	Star anise
	Swerve sweetener	Vanilla extract
	Tomato salsa	

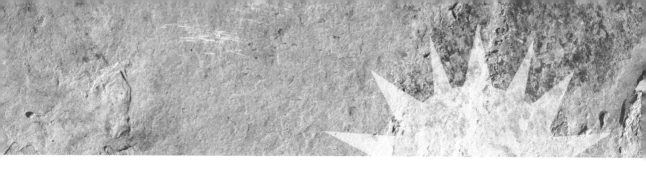

TOOLS

"Be willing to be a beginner every single morning."
—Meister Eckhart

I love simple tools. And since my kitchen is small, I try to keep only the most basic tools on hand. My favorite breakfast tools are my blender, food processor, and non-stick skillet. I feel quite fortunate to have these, since our Paleolithic ancestors were limited to an open fire, stone grinders, and cutting stones. Many of these tools can be found in a good kitchen store. Here are my suggested tools for good morning food prep.

Food processor with "S" blade and grater. KitchenAid or Cuisinart, at least eleven-cup capacity. Find them at cuisinart.com and kitchenaid.com.

Blender. Any blender will work for most recipes. There are lots of good blenders—some of them can crush ice and make mixed drinks. Some are small personal blenders for sauces and dips. However, to make coconut butter, easy nut butters, or super-creamy smoothies, you need a super-blender. The two super-blenders available are Blendtec and Vitamix.

Blendtec makes a 3-horsepower blender that is exceptionally powerful at 1,500 watts and travels easily. My Blendtec is ten years old and has never stopped or been serviced, though I use it hard three to five times a day to make smoothies, nut butters, and to grind grains. It is a joy. Consider ordering both the standard Wild-Side Jar and the small Twister container, which is great for nut butters.

Another optimal choice is the Vitamix. In this case consider also the smaller 32-ounce wet container, which can also be used for dry ingredients. Either the Blendtec or Vitamix will micronize your foods into tiny particles and thereby maximize the nutrition you'll get out of them. I consider a super-blender a necessary investment in whole food nutrition. Buy them at blendtec.com or vitamix.com.

If cost is your main issue, go ahead and start with a less expensive blender. Then when you're ready for a serious shift in nutrition and lifestyle, make the jump to a super-blender.

Small size blender or an immersion blender with cup for small quantities. I use an immersion blender, and my favorite is the Cuisinart SmartStick Handblender from cuisinart.com or amazon.com.

Hand-held grinder for grinding chia seeds and spices, such as the Krups 203 Electric Coffee and Spice Grinder available at amazon.com.

Waffle iron. Oh yes, this is a must. For those Chocolate Brownie Superfood Waffles (page 125).

Skillets, nonstick 10-inch and 8-inch. Make sure your cookware is PTFE Free. I suggest Titanium, Scanpan, Earth Pan, Thermalon by GreenPan, Cuisinart GreenGourmet, or Green Earth by Ozeri.

Baking pans. In glass or stainless steel: 9 x 13-inch, 9-inch square, 9-inch round pie pan, a 12-cup muffin tin, and a 24-cup mini-muffin tin if desired.

Bread baking pan. World Kitchen–Pyrex/Corelle 1½-qt. Pyrex loaf dish. (This is my favorite baking pan as it is nontoxic and relatively small in size, which is important for grain-free breads so they cook all the way through.)

Two baking sheets in stainless steel.
A set of nesting mixing bowls.

Digital scale that reads both pounds and metric.
English muffin rings, a set of four.
Parchment paper.
Knives. Two sizes of chef's knives, a meat knife, a sharp paring knife, a small serrated knife for removing citrus peel, and a large serrated bread knife.

BPA-free storage containers in various sizes for leftovers, muffins, quick breads, staples, and bone broth.

Ice cube trays for jams, Paleo Butter, and sauces.

Quart Mason jars (for nut butters, nut milks, and fermented veggies).

HAND TOOLS

Rubber spatula.
Spatula for a nonstick skillet.
Thin metal spatula.
Wood or silicon spatula.
Whisks in three sizes.
Citrus reamer or anything for juicing lemons.

A fine gauge strainer for dusting muffin tins with coconut flour.

Spiral vegetable slicer or mandoline slicer for zucchini noodles. I like the Saladacco Spiral Slicer, or the Paderno World Cuisine Tri-Blade Plastic Spiral Vegetable Slicer, or any stainless steel mandoline slicer. Find them all at amazon.com.

Julienne peeler for zucchini noodles. My favorite is the Kuhn Rikon Julienne Peeler from amazon.com.

Microplane grater.

Nut milk bag. Find this in any healthy grocery or at amazon.com.

WHAT EQUIPMENT IS NOT USED IN THESE RECIPES?

You won't need a microwave—I'm pretty sure it's not Paleo. Slow cookers are convenient, but I don't recommend them, as their long cooking often destroys valuable vitamins and enzymes. An espresso maker isn't necessary for perfect Cappuccino (page 98). And you won't need a bread machine to make beautiful grain-free loaves.

————

HEALTHY MENU IDEAS

"When diet is correct, medicine is of no need.
When diet is wrong, medicine is of no use."
—Ayurvedic proverb

These breakfasts are designed as make-ahead recipes to save you time, so you'll never be rushed or stumped for breakfast again. The secret is planning—with just a little thinking ahead, you can pull from the freezer for instant grab-and-go meals. I suggest you freeze leftovers and combine the recipes that you and your family love into meals. Let your imagination go. This book gives you hundreds of possibilities. Here are three weeks of sample menus to get your creative juices going. Notice how it gets easier in the last week? You have 4 days off with no breakfast cooking needed!

Day 1—Italian Baked Eggs (page 204).
Day 2—Peaches and Greens Smoothie (page 87).

Day 3—Mini Broccoli Cheese Quiches (page 219). Eat four and freeze eight.
Day 4—Southwest Frittata (page 215).
Day 5—Big Breakfast Cookies (page 157). Eat four and freeze the rest.
Day 6—Fluffy White Bread (page 55), with easy Scrambled Eggs with Cheese. Eat four slices of bread and freeze the rest.
Day 7—Wild Salmon Cakes with Sour Cream (page 233). Eat two and freeze the rest.
Day 8—Apple Cinnamon Granola (page 103) with Homemade Coconut Milk (page 35). Put the granola in a jar and refrigerate the remaining milk.
Day 9—Defrost two Mini Broccoli Quiches from day 3. Heat briefly in

the oven. Make Paleo Butter (page 45) and freeze it in an ice cube tray. Enjoy it with toasted Fluffy White Bread from day 6.

Day 10—High-Protein Kefir Berry Smoothie (page 85). Use the coconut milk you made on day 8.

Day 11—Personal Pizza for One (page 180).

Day 12—Cowboy Baked Eggs (page 203). Yum! Freeze two portions.

Day 13—Defrost Wild Salmon Cakes from day 7. Make Bacon Chili Cornbread mini muffins (page 71). Freeze twenty muffins. Spread today's muffins with Paleo Butter from day 9.

Day 14—Day off. Defrost two Big Breakfast Cookies. Enjoy with a cup of Cappuccino (page 98).

Day 15—Bacon Cauliflower Hash with Eggs (page 171). Eat half, freeze half. Enjoy it with toasted Fluffy White Bread from day 6.

Day 16—No cooking today. Apple Cinnamon Granola from day 8, with berries and homemade almond milk (page 36).

Day 17—Day off. Defrost and heat Mini Broccoli Cheese Quiches from day 3.

Day 18—Sunrise Green Smoothie (page 89).

Day 19—Day off. Defrost Wild Salmon Cakes from day 7.

Day 20—Make Old-World Seed Bread (page 59). Enjoy it with homemade almond butter (page 38). Eat two slices and freeze the rest.

Day 21—Day off. Defrost Cowboy Baked Eggs from day 12. Eat them with Bacon Chili Cornbread mini muffins from day 13 and Paleo Butter. Yum!

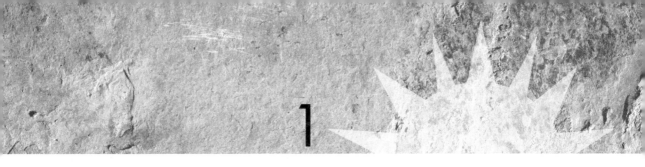

BREAKFAST STAPLES

"Simplicity is the ultimate sophistication."
—Leonardo da Vinci

When you choose a healthy diet, all your intelligence and energies come together to help you achieve your goal. These breakfast basics will assist your shift to a thriving Paleo lifestyle. Just a little planning can save enormous amounts of time and money and ensures you'll always have a healthy breakfast. If your kitchen is anything like mine, there are always changes. It's a constant revolution, ahem, *evolution* of learning new things. Consider taking these changes one step at a time at a comfortable pace for you. My rule of thumb for the past two decades is to make one change per week—discover a new ingredient, find an improved kitchen setup, learn a new technique—no matter how small. It really adds up, and in no time your healthy Paleo kitchen can be humming, convenient, and economical.

First of all, you'll save on homemade staples. Three of the best ways to reduce food spending is to make your own milks, nut butters, and coconut butter. You'll enjoy a vast improvement in flavor in just minutes a week and save bundles compared to store prices.

Coconut butter (page 33) is my #1 favorite basic, also called coconut cream and coconut manna. It's the first recipe in the book because it's a perfect grain-free flour substitute, nutrient-rich, and hypoallergenic. I use coconut butter in many of the recipes in this book—from pancakes to muffins, quiche to cheese sauces. You can buy it ready-made in stores; but, even better, you can make it yourself for a small fraction of the store price. You'll need a super-blender such as the Blendtec or VitaMix or a food processor to make coconut butter yourself, and I highly recommend the investment.

Not only will you save money, you'll save time—and improve your health while at it. Use these nutritious basics to cultivate true health. For example, Fermented Veggies (page 48) can give you a natural probiotic every morning. Nutrient-rich Homemade Bone Broth (page 47) is a great base for Egg Drop Soup (page 191) and other breakfasts.

While you're enjoying a flavorful breakfast, these basics are time-savers. Throw a handful of Homemade Bacon Bits (page 42) into your eggs. Enjoy Paleo Butter (page 45) on your morning toast. Or spread Paleo Cream Cheese (page 43) on your English Muffins (page 67). To store sauces and cheeses, freeze in ice cube trays overnight, wrapped in plastic to protect their delicate flavor. Then transfer cubes to a resealable bag for storage. Pull out a cube when you need it.

The most important factor in changing your diet is attitude. Have compassion with yourself. Take the time to stop and just notice the tough moments. Can you smile and appreciate them? This book is intended to support you to face the challenges, to restore, or maintain your health, starting with breakfast.

———————

COCONUT BUTTER

Coconut butter is a true staple ingredient. It's pure coconut meat, ground into nut butter, with a creamy, sweet taste. Sometimes called coconut cream or coconut manna, you can buy it in any healthy grocery. Or you can make it yourself for a fraction of the store price. I was amazed to discover that coconut butter, which is simply finely ground shredded coconut, can be used as a grain-free flour in recipes like Banana Bread (page 39), Pumpkin Muffins (page 150), Fluffy White Bread (page 55), or as a cheese substitute in Spicy Cheese Sauce (page 258). Coconut butter is hypoallergenic and tree nut–free; it contains one-quarter of the carbs in wheat flour or processed coconut flour.

Coconut butter is quite hard at room temperature and requires a knife to remove it in chunks from the jar. Cold, solid coconut butter is easy to measure by weight, but more difficult to accurately measure by the cup—the hard chunks just don't go into cups very well. However, softened coconut butter is more liquid, so it can be accurately measured in cups. Each recipe will give you the amount in both cups and weight, so you can choose how you want to measure it.

Store at room temperature for up to a year.

YIELD: See chart below • **EQUIPMENT:** A food processor or super-blender such as Vitamix or Blendtec (a regular blender will not work)

Pure unsweetened shredded coconut flakes

Shredded coconut	Yield in Coconut Butter
2½ cups	1 cup
3¼ cups	1¼ cups
3½ cups	1⅓ cups
3¾ cups	1½ cups
4¼ cups	1⅔ cups
4½ cups	1¾ cups
5 cups	2 cups

- Put the shredded coconut in your machine and press start. The coconut will go through different stages as it grinds—first crumbly, then grainy, then balling up like dough. Finally it becomes smooth and creamy. Just let the machine run until the oil has released

continues

and the butter is smooth. Stop and scrape the sides, tamping it down if necessary. In a super-blender, this process takes 1 to 2 minutes. In a food processor it takes longer, 5 to 10 minutes to get a smooth butter. Above all, do not worry, and do not add water.

• When it becomes smooth and creamy, pour it into a glass jar.

Tip #1: If you're making a recipe using a food processor or blender, to save time you can weigh the hard coconut butter, add it to the container, and let the machine grind it for you. If you're mixing by hand or don't have a scale, you can first soften the coconut butter by placing the jar in a bowl of very warm water for 20 to 30 minutes. Then measure out the soft butter in a cup measure and add it to your recipe.

Tip #2: I find it quicker to weigh coconut butter, rather than pressing it into a measuring cup. Each recipe gives you a choice by cup or by weight, so you can choose what's easiest for you. Here's a quick conversion chart below:

MEASURING COCONUT BUTTER		
Cups	**Grams**	**Ounces**
1 tablespoon	14 grams	1 ounce
2 tablespoons	28 grams	2 ounces
¼ cup	57 grams	4 ounces
⅓ cup	75 grams	5 ounces
½ cup	113 grams	8 ounces
⅔ cup	151 grams	11 ounces
¾ cup	170 grams	12 ounces
1 cup	227 grams	16 ounces
1¼ cups	283 grams	20 ounces
1⅓ cups	302 grams	21 ounces
1½ cups	340 grams	24 ounces
1⅔ cups	378 grams	27 ounces
1¾ cups	397 grams	28 ounces
2 cups	454 grams	32 ounces

Gluten-free	Dairy-free	Egg-free	Meat-free	Tree Nut-free	Vegan	Diabetic-friendly	Candida-friendly	High-protein	10 minutes or less
●	●	●	●	●	●	●	●		●

HOMEMADE COCONUT MILK

Quick to make and easy on the pocketbook, homemade coconut milk is creamier, tastier, and healthier than store-bought milks. It's also fresher, without the chemicals and sweeteners common in coconut beverages. Blend it in minutes from shredded coconut to use in Quiche Lorraine (page 222) or the Blueberry Orange Smoothie (page 80). Add it to crispy Apple Cinnamon Granola (page 103) or just enjoy it plain. For a nutrition boost and delicious flavor, see the High-Protein Coconut Milk variation below. You can freeze the pulp in small bags for later use or dry it in the oven at the lowest temperature for about 1½ hours. Use it in granola, or cookies instead of almond meal. Oh, and don't forget to spice up your coconut milk with the tempting flavor options like Vanilla, Spicy Chai, or Pumpkin—(page 37). It will keep in the refrigerator for 2 to 4 days. For perfect coffee creamer cubes one dose at a time, freeze it in an ice cube tray overnight, then transfer cubes to a resealable bag for up to 3 months.

YIELD: 4 cups • **EQUIPMENT:** Any blender, although a high-speed blender such as a Blendtec or Vitamix works best. A quart Mason jar is helpful.

2 cups shredded unsweetened coconut   4 cups warm filtered water

- Place the shredded coconut in the blender. In a quart Mason jar, add 2 cups cold filtered water, and 2 cups very hot water. Pour it into the blender with the coconut.

- Blend well for about a minute. Stop and allow the machine to rest. Then blend again for another minute.

- Place a nut milk bag in a saucepan and pour the blended milk into it. Lift the bag and squeeze out your creamy milk. To add flavorings, rinse the blender and pour the milk back into it. Add your favorite flavorings—see suggestions on page 37—and blend briefly. Pour into a quart glass jar. Enjoy.

VARIATION: High-Protein Coconut Milk
My favorite coconut milk is high-nutrient, protein-rich, and tastes wonderful in any recipe that calls for coconut milk. It's great on Apple Cinnamon Granola (page 103) or Flax Oatmeal with Banana (page 108). To make it, follow the previous recipe. After squeezing the milk from the bag, rinse the blender and pour the milk back into it. Add 1 scoop of your favorite protein powder. Mine is Bluebonnet Whey Protein Isolate Original. Add any flavorings desired (page 37), blend, and enjoy.

Gluten-free	Dairy-free	Egg-free	Meat-free	Tree Nut-free	Vegan	Diabetic-friendly	Candida-friendly	High-protein	10 minutes or less
●	●	●	●	●	●	●	●		●

HOMEMADE NUT MILK

Fresh nut milks are a super-easy, high-nutrition beverage and a boon for anyone on a budget. Besides being dairy-free, they're packed with healthy vitamins, minerals, and fatty acids that offer powerful health benefits, boosting mental awareness and mood. Go ahead, whip up a quick batch of this easy nut milk-just to humor me. I guarantee the creamy, real-food taste will be so superior to expensive, store-bought beverages, you'll never go back. Why pay more for imported, chemical dilutions, when you can make the real deal quicker yourself? Nut milk lasts about 3 days in the fridge.

Choose your nut. Almond milk is the most popular, with a mild flavor and high protein content. You can try rich and creamy cashew milk, or hazelnut milk with its distinctive, elegant flavor. Pumpkin seed milk is slightly sweet and nutty, whereas hemp milk is high in omega-3 fatty acids, with a subtle earthy taste.

You can make your nut milk thicker by adding more nuts or less water. To use leftover pulp, either dehydrate or bake in the oven at the lowest temperature for about 1½ hours. Use it just as you would use almond meal in flatbread, granola, or cookies. Oh, and try the irresistible nut milk flavorings on page 37—the possibilities are endless!

YIELD: 4 cups • **EQUIPMENT:** Any blender will do. You'll enjoy a creamier nut milk and a better nutritional value with a super-blender, but it is not required. Don't have a blender? Use a food processor. A quart Mason jar is helpful.

1 cup nuts, soaked if possible (page 40). Dehydrated or toasted is fine too.
4 cups filtered water

- Put the nuts into a blender. Add filtered water and blend well for about a minute. Stop and allow the machine to rest. Then blend again for another minute.

- Place a nut milk bag in a saucepan. Pour the milk into the bag. Lift the bag out and squeeze. Pour the milk into a clean glass jar (like a Mason jar).

- To add flavorings, rinse the blender, and pour the milk back into it. Choose your favorite flavorings—see options on page 37—and blend briefly.

continues

continued

VARIATION: High-Protein Nut Milk

You can make your nut milk even more nutritious by using this high-protein variation in any recipe calling for nut milk. It's yummy on Cocoa-Nutty Granola (page 104). To make it, follow the previous recipe. After squeezing the milk from the bag, rinse the blender, and pour the milk back into it. Add 1 scoop of your favorite protein powder. Mine is Bluebonnet Whey Protein Isolate Original. Add any flavorings desired (see below), blend, and enjoy.

Optional Flavorings for Nut Milk and Coconut Milk

Vanilla—Add ½ teaspoon vanilla, a pinch of unprocessed salt, 1 tablespoon sweetener

Chocolate—Add ½ teaspoon vanilla, 1 to 2 tablespoons pure cacao powder, 2 to 3 tablespoons sweetener

Cinnamon—Add ½ teaspoon vanilla, ½ teaspoon ground cinnamon, and 1 tablespoon sweetener

Mayan Chocolate—Add ½ teaspoon vanilla, 3 tablespoons pure cacao powder, 4 tablespoons brown sweetener, ½ teaspoon ground cinnamon, a pinch of ground cayenne, a pinch of unprocessed salt

Salted Caramel—Add 1 teaspoon vanilla, ⅛ teaspoon unprocessed salt, 2 tablespoons brown sweetener, ¼ teaspoon maple flavor

Very Berry—Add ½ cup berries, fresh or frozen, ½ teaspoon vanilla, 1–2 tablespoons sweetener

Spicy Chai—Add 1 teaspoon vanilla, ⅛ teaspoon unprocessed salt, 2 tablespoons brown sweetener, ½ teaspoon ground cinnamon, ¼ teaspoon ground cardamom, ⅛ teaspoon ground cloves, ¼ teaspoon ground ginger, a pinch of black pepper

Pumpkin—Add ½ cup pumpkin puree, 1 teaspoon vanilla, ¼ teaspoon maple flavor, 2 tablespoons sweetener, and 1 teaspoon pumpkin pie spice. (No pumpkin pie spice? Use ½ teaspoon cinnamon, ¼ teaspoon ground nutmeg, and a pinch each of ground cloves and ground ginger.)

Caramel Macchiato—Add 1 teaspoon vanilla, ⅛ teaspoon unprocessed salt, 2 to 4 tablespoons brown sweetener, 1 teaspoon decaffeinated coffee crystals, ¼ teaspoon maple flavor, a pinch of ground cinnamon

Gluten-free	Dairy-free	Egg-free	Meat-free	Tree Nut-free	Vegan	Diabetic-friendly	Candida-friendly	High-protein	10 minutes or less
●	●	●	●		●	●	●		●

HOMEMADE NUT BUTTER

Go beyond the peanut with these healthy, homemade nut butters. While almond butter is the most common, you can make butter with cashews, hazelnuts, and sunflower seeds. They're all concentrated protein, healthy fats, and rich taste. For best flavor and digestibility follow the instructions for Soaking and Crisping Nuts (page 40). The rest is up to your creative imagination. Try nut butters with two or more types of nut or add flavorings. How about cashew-almond butter with honey and cinnamon? The possibilities are endless. You can spread hazelnut butter on toasted English Muffins (page 67). Enjoy fresh almond butter on Old-World Seed Bread (page 59). Store covered in the refrigerator for up to a month.

YIELD: About 1 cup • **EQUIPMENT:** Any food processor or a super-blender such as a Vitamix or Blendtec

2 cups nuts, soaked and toasted if possible (page 40).
 Almonds, cashews, sunflower seeds, pecans, pumpkin seeds,
 hazelnuts, Brazil nuts, walnuts, or macadamia nuts
 (For hemp nuts, use them raw.)

OPTIONAL ADDITIONS:
2 tablespoons coconut oil or olive oil
2 teaspoons raw honey or 3 teaspoons zero-carb sweetener (see page 18 for options)
¼ teaspoon unprocessed salt
¼ teaspoon ground cinnamon

- Put the nuts in your machine and turn it on. The nuts go through different stages as they grind—first raw to crumbly, to grainy, to balling up like dough. Finally they become smooth and creamy. Just let the machine run until the oil has released and the butter is smooth. Stop and scrape the sides, tamping it down if necessary. In a super-blender, this transformation happens in 1 to 2 minutes. In a food processor it takes longer, 5 to 10 minutes to get a smooth butter. Above all, do not worry, and do not add water.

- Add optional ingredients, if desired.

- Pour into a glass jar, cover, and refrigerate.

Gluten-free	Dairy-free	Egg-free	Meat-free	Tree Nut–free	Vegan	Diabetic-friendly	Candida-friendly	High-protein	10 minutes or less
●	●	●	●		●	●	●	●	●

CHOCOLATE NUT BUTTER

A mouthwatering treat that you can make ahead in minutes, Chocolate Nut Butter tastes something like Nutella, only better—much better! Spread on your favorite toast, like Old-World Sweet Potato Bread with Pecans (page 143) or Fluffy White Bread (page 55). Store covered in the refrigerator for up to a month.

YIELD: About 1 cup

- Follow the Homemade Nut Butter recipe (page 38). When the butter has reached the desired consistency, add:

2 tablespoons raw honey or 3 tablespoons zero-carb sweetener
    (see page 18 for options)
1½ tablespoons pure cacao powder
1 teaspoon vanilla
A pinch of unprocessed salt
1 teaspoon coconut oil, if needed to thin (melt it first by putting
    the jar in a bowl of warm water)

Gluten-free	Dairy-free	Egg-free	Meat-free	Tree Nut-free	Vegan	Diabetic-friendly	Candida-friendly	High-protein	10 minutes or less
●	●	●	●		●			●	●

SOAKING AND CRISPING NUTS

Nuts are a nutrient-dense source of proteins, healthy fats, and enzymes. However, they also contain bitter coatings of enzyme inhibitors, which often irritate the lining of the intestines. Soaking neutralizes the inhibitors and reduces bitterness. Native peoples in Central America soak their nuts and seeds in seawater and then dry them. Even squirrels know how to sprout nuts by burying them in the ground! Soaking nuts is always optional (you'll see a few varieties listed below that don't require soaking). However after you become accustomed to sweet, healthy, digestible nuts, you'll never want to go back. Look for a reliable source for fresh nuts that are cultivated with care. Because nuts are high in natural oils, they can easily become rancid. Many groceries stock nuts for years without rotating or refrigerating them. Look for nuts that are rotated, refrigerated, and have a rapid turnover.

HOW TO SOAK NUTS AND SEEDS

- Soak 2 to 6 cups of shelled almonds, Brazil nuts, pecans, pumpkin seeds, sesame seeds, sunflower seeds, and walnuts in room temperature filtered water to cover with 2 teaspoons of unprocessed salt for 7 to a maximum of 24 hours. Soaking overnight is convenient for most people.

- Cashews should be soaked for no more than 6 hours, or they may become bitter.

- No need to soak hemp nuts, macadamia nuts, pine nuts, or pistachios, as these nuts are very low in phytates.

- Rinse and drain the soaked nuts. It is important to crisp or toast them within a day or they could attract mold.

continues

continued

HOW TO CRISP AND TOAST NUTS FOR STORING

Crispy Nuts

Crispy nuts are dried, but not roasted. They'll stay crunchy and tasty for months in an airtight container. Once you've soaked, drained, and rinsed the nuts or seeds, spread them in a dehydrator or glass baking pan. If you have a dehydrator, dehydrate for 12 to 24 hours at 120°F or until dry and crispy. Or you can bake them in the oven at the lowest temperature—110 to 150°F for 10 to 24 hours with the oven door cracked open, stirring from time to time. The total crisping time will depend on your dehydrator or oven and the moisture content of your nuts.

Toasted Nuts

Toasted nuts are quicker, and they have a deeper roasted flavor than crisped nuts.

After soaking your nuts, rinse and drain them well. Put the wet nuts in a parchment-lined baking pan. Toast nuts at 200 to 250°F with the oven door barely cracked open for 3 to 5 hours. Set a timer to stir them and turn the pan every 30 minutes, watching their progress. The object is to dry them completely so they're crispy all the way through. If you bake them at a higher temperature, they may toast on the outside, but be wet and soggy in the center. The total baking time will depend on the moisture level and the size of the nut.

I find it easiest to buy nuts, soak them all, and then toast or crisp them all right away, so they're always ready for snacks, nut butters, and breakfasts (and crisping or toasting many batches of nuts at once conserves energy).

> **Tip:** Taste a nut to see if they're crispy all the way through. And keep an eye on them so they don't burn.

Gluten-free	Dairy-free	Egg-free	Meat-free	Tree Nut-free	Vegan	Diabetic-friendly	Candida-friendly	High-protein	10 minutes or less
●	●	●	●		●	●	●	●	

HOMEMADE BACON BITS

Bacon bits are a flavorful addition to any Paleo dish and a huge time-saver—not to mention so much healthier than the processed, commercial bacon bits (many of which don't even include actual bacon). You'll want to sprinkle them on everything! Try them on Sweet Potato Hash with Turkey Apple Sausage (page 170) and Personal Pizza for One (page 180). Look for non-GMO, sugar-free bacon, if possible. Store in an airtight container up to 3 months.

YIELD: 1½ to 2 cups bacon bits

1 pound sliced bacon
¼ teaspoon ground black pepper

- Preheat the oven to 350°F. Get out a large baking pan with a lip to avoid spills. Cover it with parchment paper.

- Partially freeze the bacon for about 30 minutes so it is easier to cut in pieces.

- Using a sharp knife, cut bacon lengthwise into narrow strips ¼ inch wide. Rotate and cut the strips into bits ¼ inch wide. Sprinkle with black pepper.

- Bake for 20 to 25 minutes until crisp, stirring every 5 minutes. You can also fry it in a large skillet until crisp. In both cases pour off the bacon grease for later use.

- Put the bacon pieces on a parchment-covered tray in a single layer, and freeze for 30 minutes. This insures that the frozen bits will be easy to grab and sprinkle, instead of a solid mass. Then freeze them in a storage container.

Gluten-free	Dairy-free	Egg-free	Meat-free	Tree Nut-free	Vegan	Diabetic-friendly	Candida-friendly	High-protein	10 minutes or less
●	●	●		●		●		●	

PALEO CREAM CHEESE

I'd been feeling cream cheese–deprived for years—until I invented this recipe! Smooth, rich, and creamy, it's an easy spread that's quick to blend and incredibly tasty. The main ingredients are coconut butter and lemon. This "cheese" is temperature-sensitive, so it is runny when blended, spreadable at room temperature, and quite hard when chilled. Remove it from the refrigerator or freezer several hours before using, to allow it to soften to the perfect texture. Use just as you would use any cream cheese. Crumble it on the Asparagus Frittata (page 197) or spread it on Pumpernickel Rye Bread (page 61). This is easy to make ahead and freeze in a BPA-free container for up to 3 months. Thaw it for a few minutes and cut out what you need. Try the Herbed Cream Cheese variation below.

YIELD: 1½ cups • **EQUIPMENT:** A small blender or food processor

¾ cup unsweetened coconut milk, medium to thick (page 35)
2½ tablespoons lemon juice
1 teaspoon apple cider vinegar
1 teaspoon nutritional yeast
¼ heaping teaspoon unprocessed salt to taste
½ cup (113 grams) coconut butter (page 33), softened
    (place the container in a bowl of warm water)
3 tablespoons coconut oil

- Put coconut milk, lemon juice, vinegar, nutritional yeast, and salt in the blender. Blend until smooth. Add the coconut butter and blend again. Add coconut oil last and blend until smooth.

- Chill for 2 hours to thicken.

VARIATION: Herbed Cream Cheese
Follow the recipe above. When it is finished, stir in by hand a ¼ cup of finely minced fresh or dried herbs, such as basil, chives, green onions, cilantro, parsley, or dill. Serve.

Gluten-free	Dairy-free	Egg-free	Meat-free	Tree Nut-free	Vegan	Diabetic-friendly	Candida-friendly	High-protein	10 minutes or less
●	●	●	●	●	●	●	●		●

PALEO FETA CHEESE

This dairy-free cheese tastes and crumbles just like feta. Made with coconut, nutritional yeast gives it a cheese flavor, while vitamin C crystals make it tart—find them in the grocery supplements section. It's a delicious addition to Mediterranean dishes like Greek Egg "Eyes" (page 206) or Spinach and Feta Quiche (page 224). The flavor is similar to Paleo Cream Cheese, but with a salty, tart zing. Add it to eggs, veggies, or put it in sandwiches. Freeze feta cheese in an ice cube tray overnight, then transfer the cubes to a resealable bag. Or freeze in a BPA-free container for up to 3 months and crumble it into your favorite breakfasts.

YIELD: 1½ cups • **EQUIPMENT:** A small 2-cup blender or immersion blender with cup

½ cup unsweetened coconut milk, medium to thick (page 35),
  or a wee bit more if needed to blend smoothly
¾ teaspoon unprocessed salt
⅛ teaspoon black or white pepper
3 tablespoons lemon juice
1 teaspoon apple cider vinegar
½ teaspoon vitamin C crystals (optional)
2 teaspoons nutritional yeast
2 tablespoons extra-virgin olive oil
¾ cup (170 grams) Coconut Butter (page 33) softened
  (place the container in a bowl of warm water)

- Have all the ingredients at room temperature, except the coconut butter should be slightly warm, not hot, just so it is barely softened.

- In the blender, place coconut milk, salt, pepper, lemon juice, vinegar, vitamin C crystals if using, nutritional yeast, and olive oil. Blend until smooth. Add the coconut butter last and blend until smooth. It will become very thick. Add a bit more coconut milk if necessary to blend.

- Spoon into a storage container and refrigerate or freeze to firm up.

Gluten-free	Dairy-free	Egg-free	Meat-free	Tree Nut-free	Vegan	Diabetic-friendly	Candida-friendly	High-protein	10 minutes or less
●	●	●	●	●	●	●	●		●

PALEO BUTTER

Here's a fantastic buttery spread that's quick to make and 100 percent dairy-free. This spread is more delicious and much healthier than any chemical blend in the store, and see the variation below for Paleo Butter that's high in omega-3 fatty acids. Vitamin C crystals give it a cultured European flavor—find them in the grocery supplements section. They're optional, and it tastes yummy without them. Paleo Butter is perfect on your toasted English Muffins (page 67) or Sour Cream Onion Dill toast (page 65). Spread it on Bacon Chili Cornbread (page 71) or Blueberry Pancakes (page 117). It's easy to make and keep on hand—just blend it, freeze it in ice cube trays overnight, well wrapped to protect the delicate flavor. Then transfer the cubes to a resealable plastic bag for up to 3 months, and pull out a cube when you want one.

YIELD: 1⅛ cups • **EQUIPMENT:** A blender or food processor makes it easier but is not required

¾ cup unrefined coconut oil, melted (place the jar in a bowl of warm water)
¼ cup extra-virgin olive oil
¼ teaspoon finely ground unprocessed salt
¼ teaspoon vitamin C crystals (optional)

- Place all the ingredients in the blender and blend well. If you're mixing by hand, simply whisk the ingredients together briskly until smooth and well combined.

- Pour into an ice cube tray, wrap, and freeze overnight. Then transfer to a resealable freezer bag.

VARIATION: Paleo Omega-3 Butter
Enhance the nutritional profile of your butter with flax oil. It gives you a high omega-3 shot in the arm, with a mild flavor that's hardly noticeable. Flaxseed oil contains essential fatty acids that protect cell membranes, build intestinal health, and reduce the risk of heart disease. Flax oil can be damaged by heating, so this is for spreading only, not for cooking.

Follow the recipe above, adding 2 tablespoons extra-virgin flax oil to the blender.

Gluten-free	Dairy-free	Egg-free	Meat-free	Tree Nut-free	Vegan	Diabetic-friendly	Candida-friendly	High-protein	10 minutes or less
●	●	●	●	●	●	●	●		●

PERFECT COCONUT PIE CRUST

This amazing pie crust tastes deliciously crispy and rolls out beautifully. The secret ingredients are coconut butter and chia seeds. This crust is ideal for Quiche Lorraine (page 222) or Bacon Zucchini Quiche (page 221). It is important to use standard-size large eggs, about 55 grams each out of the shell. If your eggs are smaller, your dough will be thicker. If your eggs are jumbo, the dough will be too runny. To resolve this you can either weigh the eggs, or adjust the other ingredients—see instructions below. Prebaking this crust is optional. For very moist quiches, prebaking helps to avoid a soggy crust that breaks. However, if your quiche has a more solid bottom layer of veggies and meat, there's no need to prebake.

YIELD: One 9-inch pie crust • **EQUIPMENT:** A food processor is helpful but not required

1⅓ cups (302 grams) Coconut Butter (page 33); if mixing by hand, soften butter by placing the container in a bowl of warm water

1½ tablespoons ground white chia seeds

¼ heaping teaspoon unprocessed salt

2 large eggs (110 grams total)

1 to 2 tablespoons coconut flour, to thicken if necessary

- Preheat the oven to 300°F if you plan to prebake. Get out a 9-inch pie pan. In a food processor or mixing bowl, add coconut butter, chia seeds, salt, and eggs. Mix well until the dough is smooth. Then refrigerate the dough in the container for 15 minutes to allow it to firm up.

- Check the dough consistency. It should be very thick and pliable. If it's too wet to roll, you can knead it with a tablespoon or two of coconut flour. If it is too thick to roll, beat a fresh egg and add it in increments until the dough is thick enough to press into a pie pan.

- Shape the dough into a ball. You can press it into a 9-inch pie pan with your fingers. Or you can use a rolling pin: Roll it between two pieces of parchment paper into a disk about ⅛ inch thick, and 1 inch larger than your pie pan all around. Dust with coconut flour to prevent sticking to the parchment paper. Remove the top sheet of paper. Flip the bottom paper and rolled dough over onto your pie pan and gently peel away the paper. Repair any rips and flute the edges if you wish. If you're pressing the dough into the pan with your fingers, start with a ball of dough in the center of the pie pan. Spread it with your fingers toward the edges, up the sides, and flute the edges if desired.

- If prebaking, bake for 10 to 15 minutes. Then add your filling.

Gluten-free	Dairy-free	Egg-free	Meat-free	Tree Nut-free	Vegan	Diabetic-friendly	Candida-friendly	High-protein	10 minutes or less
●	●		●	●		●	●		

HOMEMADE BONE BROTH

When you're feeling weak and tired, broth is the #1 best cure. Homemade bone broth tastes rich and satisfying, and it's surprisingly easy to simmer overnight or while you do other things. Since bone tissue is alive, it has an off-the-charts nutritional profile and cooks like an organ, so the longer it is simmered, the more nutritious the broth becomes. The best bones to use are beef tail bones, long bones, and knuckles sliced crossways, and any chicken bones, especially feet. Ask your grocer and you'll discover your favorite bones. Look for organic or grass-fed, grass-finished meats. Make ahead and freeze it in BPA-free containers for up to 6 months. Use in soups such as Pho Ga, Vietnamese Chicken Soup (page 192), Egg Drop Soup (page 191), and Zoodle Soup (page 193). Enjoy a cup of broth as a pick-me-up instead of coffee or tea. Vary the recipe as you like.

YIELD: 3 quarts • **EQUIPMENT:** Large soup pot, medium soup pot, and a large colander or strainer

4 pounds bones
2 carrots, coarsely cut with peels
2 stalks celery, coarsely cut
1 onion, peeled and halved
3 cloves garlic, smashed
1 teaspoon black peppercorns

1 to 2 tablespoons apple cider vinegar
3 bay leaves
2 teaspoons unprocessed salt
½ bunch parsley with stems
1 gallon filtered water or more to fill pot

- Put the ingredients in the large pot and add filtered water. Heat on high until it barely begins to boil.

- Just before it goes into a full rolling boil, turn the heat down. Use a large flat spoon to skim off the surface foam, which is better to remove.

- Cover and simmer on very low heat from 8 to 72 hours. When finished, the broth will be rich and flavorful. The bones will be disintegrating. Allow to cool and strain it into another pot.

- The strained broth will be beautiful and clear with a layer of liquid fat on the top.

- Chill it in the pot 4 hours or overnight. Then with a large flat spoon, scrape the fat off the top. Put the fat in a glass jar to use as a cooking fat. Oh, and pour yourself a delicious cup of broth right now. Freeze the rest for a rainy day.

Gluten-free	Dairy-free	Egg-free	Meat-free	Tree Nut-free	Vegan	Diabetic-friendly	Candida-friendly	High-protein	10 minutes or less
●	●	●		●		●	●	●	

FERMENTED VEGGIES

The easiest and healthiest make-ahead recipe you can prepare, fermented veggies are a natural probiotic that build healthy intestinal flora. And since the immune system depends on friendly bacteria in the gut, this is central to your health each day. Have fun experimenting with different vegetables, low-sugar fruits, flavors, and color combinations. Store in the refrigerator for several months and serve it as a side dish with every meal. These veggies taste great with Sweet Potato Hash with Turkey Apple Sausage (page 170) or Portobello Scramble (page 211).

YIELD: 1 quart • **EQUIPMENT NEEDED:** A food processor or blender makes it super-easy but is not required; two 1-quart glass jars with lids

3 cups vegetables—any vegetable you have! The best include cabbage, beet, carrot, daikon, broccoli, cucumber, onion, green beans, kale, chard, zucchini, wild greens, ginger, cilantro, parsley (stems and all), watercress, garlic, ginger, black pepper, soaked seaweed, Granny Smith apple

½ teaspoon unprocessed salt (optional)

1 to 2 cups filtered water

- Shred or chop your veggies: Use a food processor (grater or S-blade), a super-blender, or grate and chop them by hand. It doesn't matter how large they are. Small particles will ferment a bit faster. Stir in the salt, if using.

- Pack the veggies tightly into a quart jar (like a Mason jar). Press them down tight to remove any air pockets. I use a drinking glass as a press.

- Add water so it is 1 inch higher than the veggies. Some people like to cover them with a big cabbage leaf or a slice of cabbage rind. The idea is to weigh them down to keep the veggies under the surface of the liquid. Leave an inch of empty space above the water. Some people like to add a few teaspoons of liquid from another batch of fermented veggies as a starter—this is optional.

continues

continued

- Screw the lid on the jar tightly and leave in a dark cupboard. Fermentation takes 4 to 14 days depending on the temperature. In the summer 4 to 7 days, wintertime about 2 weeks. The ideal temperature is 68 to 75 °F. If the veggies rise above the water, push them back down to keep them submerged. To check if it's ready, taste it with a clean spoon. When finished, have a big serving and store the rest in the refrigerator. It'll keep for 6 months or more.

Tip: Yes, it can happen, rarely, that unfriendly bacteria gets in. You'll know immediately, as the veggies will be brownish, slimy, and inedible.

Gluten-free	Dairy-free	Egg-free	Meat-free	Tree Nut-free	Vegan	Diabetic-friendly	Candida-friendly	High-protein	10 minutes or less
●	●	●	●	●	●	●	●		

2

SAVORY BREADS

"What nicer thing can you do for somebody than make them breakfast?"
—Anthony Bourdain

Starting the Paleo diet and avoiding gluten and grains does *not* mean giving up your favorite breads. There is no deprivation here. On the contrary, the textures of these breads and the variety of flavors defy the very idea of "limitation." This chapter gives you eighteen scrumptious bread recipes from Almond Sandwich Bread (page 53) to Rosemary Olive Bread (page 63). With so many choices in Paleo-friendly breads, you can enjoy sandwiches and toast once again. Even better, since they're grain-free, they're much lower in carbs than their refined counterparts.

Let's take a moment to define grains and gluten. Grains are grasses that are cultivated for their seeds, such as wheat and corn. Gluten is a sticky protein found in some grains, which makes baked goods hold together, and which many people find indigestible. Gluten is found primarily in wheat, rye, and barley grains. The good news is the Paleo diet is grain-free, so it is 100 percent gluten-free as well. Hooray!

We've all tried gluten-free, grain-free bread that tastes like tree bark and falls apart in your hands. The good news is that you can make luscious, grain-free breads, and the secret ingredient is chia seeds. Chia seeds are a high-protein superfood and a wonderful addition to baked goods. They absorb liquid, creating a viscous mixture that mimics the flavor and consistency of wheat dough. Chia seeds act as a binder so the loaves hold together like traditional breads. I use white chia seeds to imitate the light color of grains—and presto! You've got sliced bread.

Another secret ingredient in grain-free bread is nut butter. These breads are unbelievably soft and feather-light. For example, Fluffy White Bread (page 55) and Fluffy Almond Butter Bread (page 54) are perfect for your morning toast. The easy English Muffins (page 67) get their pleasing texture in part from coconut butter.

None of these breads use yeast. Instead they're leavened with the age-old combination of baking soda and live vinegar. So you don't have to wait 30 to 60 minutes for the dough to rise—just put it right in the oven and bake. It is best to put these breads in the oven immediately on mixing, so the rising action happens there, and they'll come out as light and fluffy as possible. If you delay baking, your breads may be denser and harder. For a pleasant crunch to your bread, you can add pumpkin seeds, sesame seeds, walnuts, almonds, and so on. However, don't use sunflower seeds or sunflower seed butter in quick breads. The natural acid in sunflower seeds reacts to baking soda and will turn your bread green, as I discovered to my great surprise. This is the only caveat to breads with baking soda. However if you substitute yeast for baking soda and vinegar, your bread will come out beautifully and will not react to sunflower seeds.

These breads are ideal to make ahead and freeze, so you can pull out a slice for a quick breakfast. To store, slice the bread. Cut parchment paper into small squares and place between each slice. Put in a labeled freezer bag. For tortillas and flatbreads, freeze them on a paper plate with parchment paper between each slice, in a freezer bag.

There are so many new techniques waiting to be discovered. Let your curiosity and imagination go wild. It's more than fun—being creative makes it easier to surmount the challenges in your new diet.

———————

ALMOND SANDWICH BREAD

If you can fry an egg, you can make bread. This is a simple, old-world sandwich bread, and the first recipe where I discovered the magic of chia seeds. It has a full-bodied flavor and a pleasingly dense texture that slices and toasts beautifully. Spread it with Paleo Butter (page 45), or Orange Marmalade (page 245). Freeze it with parchment paper between the slices for a quick toast or sandwich in the morning.

YIELD: One 7 x 3-inch loaf or one 9 x 5-inch loaf • **EQUIPMENT:** A food processor is helpful but not required

	Small loaf	Large loaf
	7 x 3-inch	**9 x 5-inch**
Eggs	3 large eggs (165 grams)	6 large eggs (330 grams)
White chia seeds, ground	¼ cup	½ cup
Apple cider vinegar	2 teaspoons	4 teaspoons
Coconut oil, melted	2 tablespoons	¼ cup
Almond meal	1 ¼ cups or a bit more if needed	2 ½ cups or a bit more if needed
Baking soda	⅜ teaspoon (a bit less than ½ teaspoon)	¾ teaspoon
Unprocessed salt	⅜ teaspoon (a bit less than ½ teaspoon)	¾ teaspoon

- Preheat the oven to 350°F. Choose your loaf size—small or large. Line the pan with parchment paper so it hangs over the sides as handles.

- Crack the eggs into a small mixing bowl. Stir in the chia seeds, vinegar, and coconut oil. Allow the mixture to sit for at least 15 minutes to thicken.

- In a mixing bowl or food processor, mix together the dry ingredients: almond meal, baking soda, and salt.

- Add the egg mixture and mix well. If the dough seems too loose, add a bit more almond meal until the dough is the texture of thick cooked oatmeal.

- Bake a 7 x 3-inch loaf for 30 to 35 minutes, a 9 x 5-inch loaf for 45 to 50 minutes, or until a toothpick comes out clean. Cool before slicing.

Gluten-free	Dairy-free	Egg-free	Meat-free	Tree Nut-free	Vegan	Diabetic-friendly	Candida-friendly	High-protein	10 minutes or less
●	●		●			●	●	●	

FLUFFY ALMOND BUTTER BREAD

This bread is so easy you won't believe it until you try it. Mix it in one step in 5 minutes, bake, slice, and eat. While it's baking your kitchen will be filled with the delicious aroma of toasted almonds. It rises, slices, and toasts beautifully, just like its sister recipe, Fluffy White Bread (page 55). Make this high-protein bread with any nut butter, except sunflower seed butter. It tastes heavenly with Blueberry Chia Jam (page 244) or toasted with Wild Salmon Cauliflower Hash (page 174). Freeze it with parchment paper between the slices, and you'll have a blank palette for any breakfast you'd like to make with it.

YIELD: One 7 x 3-inch loaf or one 9 x 5-inch loaf • **EQUIPMENT:** A food processor is helpful but not required

	Small loaf	Large loaf
	7 x 3-inch	**9 x 5-inch**
Eggs at room temperature	3 large eggs (165 grams)	6 large eggs (330 grams)
Roasted almond butter (page 38)	1 cup	2 cups
Unprocessed salt	⅜ teaspoon	¾ teaspoon
Baking soda	½ teaspoon	1 teaspoon
Apple cider vinegar	1 tablespoon	2 tablespoons

- Preheat the oven to 350°F. Choose your loaf size—small or large. Line the pan with parchment paper so it hangs over the sides as handles.

- In a large food processor or mixing bowl, place the eggs, almond butter, salt, and baking soda. Mix until smooth.

- Add the vinegar and mix very well. The batter should be the texture of smooth pancake batter. Pour the dough into the baking pan.

- Bake a 7 x 3-inch loaf for 30 to 35 minutes, a 9 x 5-inch loaf for 40 to 50 minutes, or until a toothpick comes out clean. Cool before slicing.

Gluten-free	Dairy-free	Egg-free	Meat-free	Tree Nut–free	Vegan	Diabetic-friendly	Candida-friendly	High-protein	10 minutes or less
●	●		●			●	●	●	

FLUFFY WHITE BREAD

My taste-testers call this Paleo Wonder Bread, because it's soft and perfectly white. It slices and toasts beautifully. A sandwich bread with only five ingredients, it is one of the easiest recipes in the book. And there is absolutely no flour, believe it or not! Miraculously, it rises during baking to make a fluffy, light loaf that's loaded with coconut nutrition. If you use whole eggs, it will be golden yellow color. If you use egg whites or egg white powder (see Ingredients, page 17), it will be pure white. If you're using a food processor, it's not necessary to soften the coconut butter—just add it in chunks and let the machine do your work. If you're mixing by hand, you'll need to soften the coconut butter first (place the container in a bowl of warm water). Make this bread with any nut butter, except not sunflower seed butter. This is absolutely yummy with homemade almond butter (page 38) or Orange Marmalade (page 245). See the variation below for Cinnamon Swirl Bread, used for the amazing Cinnamon Swirl French Toast (page 131). You can freeze this bread in a plastic bag with parchment paper between the slices.

YIELD: One 7 x 3-inch loaf or one 9 x 5-inch loaf • **EQUIPMENT:** A food processor is helpful but not required

	Small loaf	**Large loaf**
	7 x 3-inch	**9 x 5-inch**
Coconut Butter (page 33)	1 cup (227 grams)	2 cups (454 grams)
Egg whites, room temperature	6 egg whites	12 egg whites
Or	3 whole large eggs (165 grams)	6 whole large eggs (330 grams)
Or	3 tablespoons egg white powder and 9 tablespoons lukewarm filtered water	6 tablespoons egg white powder and 1 cup + 2 tablespoons lukewarm filtered water
Unprocessed salt	⅜ teaspoon (a bit less than ½ teaspoon)	¾ teaspoon
Baking soda	½ teaspoon	1 teaspoon
Apple cider vinegar	1 tablespoon	2 tablespoons

continues

- Preheat the oven to 350°F. Choose your loaf size—small or large. Line the pan with parchment paper so it hangs over the sides as handles.

- In a food processor or mixing bowl, place the coconut butter, egg whites (or whole eggs or egg white powder and water), salt, and baking soda. Mix until smooth.

- Add the vinegar and mix well. The dough will be the consistency of pancake batter. Pour the dough into the baking pan.

- Bake a 7 x 3-inch loaf for 30 to 35 minutes, a 9 x 5-inch loaf for 40 to 50 minutes, or until a toothpick comes out clean. Cool before slicing.

VARIATION: Cinnamon Swirl Bread

Mix cinnamon swirl: For a 7 x 3-inch pan: Stir together 2 tablespoons sweetener (see page 18) with 1 tablespoon ground cinnamon. For a 9 x 5-inch pan, stir together ¼ cup sugar with 2 tablespoons cinnamon. Follow the recipe above. Pour half of the batter into the pan. Sprinkle generously with half the cinnamon sugar mixture. Repeat with the second half of the batter, sprinkling the rest of the cinnamon mixture on top. Use a table knife or a small spatula to make swirls and spirals in circular motions in the batter, to marble it. Bake as directed.

Gluten-free	Dairy-free	Egg-free	Meat-free	Tree Nut-free	Vegan	Diabetic-friendly	Candida-friendly	High-protein	10 minutes or less
●	●		●	●		●	●		

BLACK RUSSIAN SUPERFOOD CHOCOLATE MANNA BREAD

This is a rich, old-world loaf that recalls the dense, pungent flavor of Russian black bread. Many unusual ingredients—such as seaweed, green powder, cacao, fennel seed, and coffee powder—serve to enhance the authentic flavor. With all these superfoods, you'll be sure that every slice is a luscious, nutrient-dense meal. This hearty flavor blends beautifully with Paleo Cream Cheese (page 43).

YIELD: Two 4.5 x 2.5-inch mini loaves or one 7 x 3-inch loaf • **EQUIPMENT:** A food processor or blender is helpful but not required

3 large eggs
¼ cup black chia seeds, ground
2 tablespoons dried hiziki or wakame seaweed, crushed
2 tablespoons apple cider vinegar
3 tablespoons raw honey or 4 tablespoons zero-carb sweetener
   (see page 18 for options)
¼ cup coconut oil
1¼ cups almond meal
½ teaspoon baking soda
½ teaspoon unprocessed salt
3 tablespoons pure cacao powder
1 tablespoon fennel seed, powdered or well crushed
1 tablespoon nutritional yeast
2 teaspoons your favorite green powder
2 tablespoons onion flakes
1½ teaspoons decaffeinated coffee powder (optional)
¼ cup hemp nuts
3 tablespoons pumpkin seeds

• Preheat the oven to 350°F. Line the pan with parchment paper so it hangs over the sides as handles.

• In a food processor, blender, or large mixing bowl, place the eggs, chia seeds, seaweed, vinegar, honey or sweetener, and coconut oil. Mix well and allow the mixture to sit at least 15 minutes to thicken.

continues

- In a mixing bowl whisk together the almond meal, baking soda, salt, cacao, fennel seed, nutritional yeast, green powder, onion flakes, and coffee powder, if using. Mix well.

- Add the dry ingredients to the egg mixture in the food processor or mixing bowl. Mix until the dough is the texture of thick cooked oatmeal. Pulse in, or stir in the hemp nuts and pumpkin seeds.

- Spoon the dough into the baking pans. Bake the mini loaves for 20 to 22 minutes, a 7 x 3-inch pan the 30 to 35 minutes, or until a toothpick comes out clean. Cool before slicing.

Gluten-free	Dairy-free	Egg-free	Meat-free	Tree Nut–free	Vegan	Diabetic-friendly	Candida-friendly	High-protein	10 minutes or less
●	●		●					●	

OLD-WORLD SEED BREAD

This European-style nut and seed bread is delightfully crunchy—the perfect base for sandwiches. Easy to make, nutritious, and yeast-free, you can make it ahead and freeze with parchment paper between the slices. It's super-tasty toasted with Blueberry Chia Jam (page 244), Orange Marmalade (page 245), or Homemade Nut Butter (page 38).

YIELD: One 7 x 3-inch loaf or one 9 x 5-inch loaf • **EQUIPMENT:** A food processor is helpful but not required

	Small loaf	Large loaf
	7 x 3-inch	**9 x 5-inch**
Eggs	3 large eggs (165 grams)	6 large eggs (330 grams)
White chia seeds, ground	¼ cup	½ cup
Apple cider vinegar	1 tablespoon	2 tablespoons
Almond meal	1⅓ cups, or a bit more if needed	2½ cups, or a bit more if needed
Baking soda	½ teaspoon	1 teaspoon
Unprocessed salt	⅜ teaspoon (a bit less than ½ teaspoon)	¾ teaspoon
Almond butter (page 38)	2 tablespoons	¼ cup
Pumpkin seeds	¼ cup	½ cup
Sesame seeds	2 tablespoons	¼ cup
Seeds for crust, such as sesame, pumpkin, or sunflower	1 tablespoon	2 tablespoons

continues

- Preheat the oven to 350°F. Choose your loaf size—small or large. Line the pan with parchment paper so it hangs over the sides as handles.

- Crack the eggs into a small bowl. Stir in chia seeds and vinegar. Allow the mixture to sit for at least 15 minutes to thicken.

- In a mixing bowl or food processor, mix together the almond meal, baking soda, and salt.

- Add the almond butter and egg mixture. Mix well. If the dough seems too loose, add a bit more almond meal.

- Pulse or stir in pumpkin seeds and sesame seeds briefly until just mixed. The dough will be the consistency of thick cooked oatmeal.

- Press the dough into the baking pan.

- Sprinkle or spray the top with lukewarm water. Sprinkle seeds on top. Sprinkle or spray a bit more water over it again, and press seeds in gently so they'll stick.

- Bake a 7 x 3-inch loaf for 30 to 35 minutes, a 9 x 5-inch loaf for 45 to 50 minutes, or until a toothpick comes out clean. Cool before slicing.

Gluten-free	Dairy-free	Egg-free	Meat-free	Tree Nut–free	Vegan	Diabetic-friendly	Candida-friendly	High-protein	10 minutes or less
●	●		●			●	●	●	

PUMPERNICKEL RYE BREAD

If you're a fan of authentic old-world breads, you'll love the subtle flavors of this dark rye loaf. One bite transports me to Eastern Europe. It is pleasantly dense with subtle hints of fennel, caraway, and pumpkin seeds. It slices and toasts beautifully—and is loaded with whole-food nutrition. Sweetening is optional—I suggest a bit of raw honey or half brown sweetener. This bread is even tastier toasted and spread with Paleo Cream Cheese (page 43) or Paleo Butter (page 45). Freeze in an airtight container with parchment paper between the slices.

YIELD: One 7 x 3-inch loaf or one 9 x 5-inch loaf • **EQUIPMENT:** A food processor is helpful but not required

	Small loaf	Large loaf
	7 x 3-inch	**9 x 5-inch**
Eggs	3 large eggs (165 grams)	6 large eggs (330 grams)
Black chia seeds, ground	¼ cup	½ cup
Apple cider vinegar	1 tablespoon	2 tablespoons
Coconut oil, softened	3 tablespoons	6 tablespoons
Sweeten to taste: See options on page 18	1½ tablespoons	3 tablespoons
Almond meal	1¼ cups, or a bit more if needed	2¼ cups, or a bit more if needed
Baking soda	¾ teaspoon	1½ teaspoons
Unprocessed salt	⅜ teaspoon	¾ teaspoon
Carob powder	3 tablespoons	6 tablespoons
Nutritional yeast	1 tablespoon	2 tablespoons
Fennel seed, ground or crushed	1 tablespoon	2 tablespoons
Whole caraway seeds	1 tablespoon	2 tablespoons
Pumpkin seeds	¼ cup	½ cup

continues

- Preheat the oven to 350°F. Choose your loaf size—small or large. Line the pan with parchment paper so it hangs over the sides as handles.

- Crack the eggs into a food processor or mixing bowl. Stir in the chia seeds, vinegar, coconut oil, and sweetener. Allow the mixture to sit for at least 15 minutes to thicken.

- In a separate large mixing bowl, whisk together the almond meal, baking soda, salt, carob, nutritional yeast, fennel, caraway, and pumpkin seeds. Then add it to the egg mixture and process well. If the dough seems too loose, add a bit more almond meal. The dough should be about the consistency of thick cooked oatmeal.

- Place the dough in the parchment lined pan. Bake a 7 x 3-inch loaf for 30 to 35 minutes, a 9 x 5-inch loaf for 45 to 50 minutes, or until a toothpick comes out clean. Cool before slicing.

Tip: To grind whole fennel seed, use a hand-held grinder or a mortar and pestle.

Gluten-free	Dairy-free	Egg-free	Meat-free	Tree Nut-free	Vegan	Diabetic-friendly	Candida-friendly	High-protein	10 minutes or less
●	●		●			●	●	●	

ROSEMARY OLIVE BREAD

A rich, full-bodied, Mediterranean-style bread with amazing flavor and texture—you can taste the olive oil and black pepper in every savory bite. I prefer it with honey, which is optional; or you can use the same amount of zero-carb sweetener (page 18). This is scrumptious with Paleo Feta Cheese (page 44), Paleo Butter (page 45), and Italian Baked Eggs (page 204). Or you can keep it simple and just dip in olive oil. It slices and freezes well, so you can pull it out and toast it for a super-quick breakfast.

YIELD: One 7 x 3-inch loaf or one 9 x 5-inch loaf • **EQUIPMENT:** A food processor is helpful but not required

	Small loaf	Large loaf
	7 x 3-inch	**9 x 5-inch**
Eggs	3 large eggs (165 grams)	6 large eggs (330 grams)
White chia seeds, ground	¼ cup	½ cup
Apple cider vinegar	2 teaspoons	4 teaspoons
Olive oil	3 tablespoons	6 tablespoons
Raw honey (optional)	2 to 3 tablespoons	4 to 6 tablespoons
Almond meal	1¼ cups, or a bit more if needed	2½ cups, or a bit more if needed
Baking soda	⅜ teaspoon (a bit less than ½ teaspoon)	¾ teaspoon
Unprocessed salt	⅜ teaspoon (a bit less than ½ teaspoon)	¾ teaspoon
Black pepper, ground	⅛ teaspoon	¼ teaspoon
Rosemary leaves, crushed	1 tablespoon	2 tablespoons
Pecans, chopped and toasted	3 tablespoons	6 tablespoons
Kalamata olives	6 tablespoons	¾ cup

continues

- Preheat the oven to 350°F. Choose your loaf size—small or large. Line the pan with parchment paper so it hangs over the sides as handles.

- Crack the eggs into a mixing bowl. Stir in chia seeds, vinegar, olive oil, and honey, if using. Allow the mixture to sit for at least 15 minutes to thicken.

- In a mixing bowl or food processor, mix together the almond meal, baking soda, salt, pepper, and rosemary.

- Add the egg mixture and mix well.

- Pulse in the pecans and olives briefly. The dough should be the consistency of thick, cooked oatmeal.

- Pour into the pan and bake a 7 x 3-inch loaf for 30 to 35 minutes, a 9 x 5-inch loaf for 45 to 50 minutes, or until a toothpick comes out clean. Cool before slicing.

Gluten-free	Dairy-free	Egg-free	Meat-free	Tree Nut-free	Vegan	Diabetic-friendly	Candida-friendly	High-protein	10 minutes or less
●	●		●			●	●	●	

SOUR CREAM ONION DILL BREAD

I fell in love with this traditional old-world bread while working at the original Rudi's Bakery in Bloomington, Indiana, in 1973. When it bakes it fills the air with a magical savory aroma of dill and sour cream. This dairy-free, grain-free adaptation is every bit as flavorful—and healthier! It's even tastier with Paleo Cream Cheese (page 43) or Paleo Butter (page 45). Freeze it with parchment paper between the slices so you can enjoy it for many breakfasts; it goes wonderfully with omelets or frittatas.

YIELD: One 7 x 3-inch loaf or one 9 x 5-inch loaf • **EQUIPMENT:** A food processor is helpful but not required

	Small loaf	Large loaf
	7 x 3-inch	**9 x 5-inch**
Eggs	3 large eggs (165 grams)	6 large eggs (330 grams)
White chia seeds, ground	¼ cup	½ cup
Apple cider vinegar	2 teaspoons	4 teaspoons
Lemon juice	2 teaspoons	4 teaspoons
Coconut oil, softened	2 tablespoons	¼ cup
Almond meal	1¼ cups, or a bit more if needed	2½ cups, or a bit more if needed
Baking soda	⅜ teaspoon (a bit less than ½ teaspoon)	¾ teaspoon
Unprocessed salt	⅜ teaspoon (a bit less than ½ teaspoon)	¾ teaspoon
Onion flakes	3 tablespoons	6 tablespoons
Nutritional yeast	1½ teaspoons	1 tablespoon
Chopped dill	3 tablespoons	6 tablespoons

continues

continued

- Preheat the oven to 350°F. Choose your loaf size—small or large. Line the pan with parchment paper so it hangs over the sides as handles.

- Crack the eggs into a mixing bowl. Stir in chia seeds, vinegar, lemon juice, and coconut oil. Allow the mixture to sit for at least 15 minutes to thicken.

- In a mixing bowl or food processor, mix together the almond meal, baking soda, salt, onion flakes, and nutritional yeast.

- Add the egg mixture and mix well. The dough will be the consistency of thick cooked oatmeal. Add the dill and mix very briefly.

- Pour into the pan and bake a 7 x 3-inch loaf for 30 to 35 minutes, a 9 x 5-inch loaf for 45 to 50 minutes, or until a toothpick comes out clean. Cool before slicing.

Gluten-free	Dairy-free	Egg-free	Meat-free	Tree Nut-free	Vegan	Diabetic-friendly	Candida-friendly	High-protein	10 minutes or less
●	●		●			●	●	●	

ENGLISH MUFFINS

These classic English Muffins are so easy and authentic, you'll want to make—and eat—them every day. They look just like store-bought muffins—dense, fluffy, and white. The flavor is mild, with a hint of coconut. For white muffins, use egg whites or egg white powder (see Ingredients, page 17). For golden muffins, use whole eggs. Toast these English Muffins and spread them with Paleo Butter (page 45) or Blueberry Chia Jam (page 244). Freeze them in an airtight bag for quick and easy Eggs Benedict (page 208) or Egg Sandwich Made Easy (page 207).

YIELD: Four English muffins • **EQUIPMENT:** A food processor is useful but not required. A set of four English muffin rings.

5 egg whites at room temperature, or 2½ whole eggs, or 2½ tablespoons pure egg white powder in 7 tablespoons filtered water at body temperature

¾ cup (170 grams) Coconut Butter (page 33); if mixing by hand, soften butter by placing the container in a bowl of warm water

¼ teaspoon unprocessed salt

⅜ teaspoon baking soda (a little less than ½ teaspoon)

¾ tablespoon apple cider vinegar

- Preheat the oven to 350°F. Line a baking sheet with lightly greased parchment paper and place four English muffin rings on top.

- In a food processor or mixing bowl, place the egg whites, coconut butter, salt, and baking soda. Mix until smooth.

- Add the vinegar and mix very well—this begins the rising action. The batter should be about the consistency of thick pancake batter. Working quickly, use a scant ⅓ cup measure to divide the batter evenly between the four rings, smoothing the top flat. Press the rings down gently so the batter doesn't leak underneath.

- Bake for 11 to 13 minutes, until barely colored on the top. Cool on a rack for 15 minutes. Slice them all with a serrated knife.

Gluten-free	Dairy-free	Egg-free	Meat-free	Tree Nut–free	Vegan	Diabetic-friendly	Candida-friendly	High-protein	10 minutes or less
●	●		●	●		●	●		

BAKING POWDER BISCUITS

These easy drop biscuits bake up tender and golden brown in just a few minutes, perfect for Biscuits and Gravy (page 176) or simply spread hot biscuits with honey or Blueberry Chia Jam (page 244). Store them individually wrapped in resealable bags and reheat in an oven or a toaster oven.

YIELD: Nine 2-inch biscuits • **EQUIPMENT:** A food processor is helpful but not required

1¼ cups almond meal
½ cup arrowroot flour
½ teaspoon unprocessed salt
½ teaspoon baking powder
¼ teaspoon nutritional yeast (optional)
2 tablespoons cold coconut oil
1 large egg
2 tablespoons filtered water, coconut milk (page 35),
    or almond milk (page 36) (or a bit more if necessary)

- Preheat the oven to 350°F. Line a baking sheet with parchment paper.

- In a food processor or large mixing bowl, mix together the almond meal, arrowroot, salt, baking powder, and nutritional yeast, if using.

- Add the coconut oil and process. If working by hand, use a pastry cutter or two knives to cut the flour mixture into small pieces. In both cases, mix until it is in coarse crumbs.

- Add the egg and water or milk to the processor and process very briefly. Don't overmix. These are kind of rustic so a few lumps are okay.

- Drop balls of batter roughly 1½ inches in diameter onto the baking sheet, pressing them down a bit so they're flat on top and about 2 inches wide.

- Bake for 14 to 18 minutes. They won't exactly brown, but they will turn golden on the edges. Enjoy hot!

Gluten-free	Dairy-free	Egg-free	Meat-free	Tree Nut-free	Vegan	Diabetic-friendly	Candida-friendly	High-protein	10 minutes or less
●	●		●			●	●	●	

CHILI CHEESE BISCUITS

These spicy drop biscuits have a Southwest cheese flavor from lemon, nutritional yeast, onion flakes, and chili powder. The surprise superfood ingredient is—goji berries! Although optional, they add a pleasant touch of color and sweetness to an otherwise savory biscuit. Try them with zesty Chipotle Butter (page 250) or Paleo Butter (page 45). Freeze individually in resealable bags and reheat in an oven or a toaster oven.

YIELD: Twelve to fourteen 2-inch biscuits • **EQUIPMENT:** A food processor is helpful but not required

¾ cup almond meal
½ cup arrowroot flour
1 teaspoon unprocessed salt
½ teaspoon baking powder
1 tablespoon nutritional yeast
1 tablespoon chili powder
2 tablespoons lemon or lime juice

1 large egg
⅓ cup (75 grams) Coconut Butter (page 33); if mixing by hand, soften butter by placing the container in a bowl of warm water
2 tablespoons filtered water
2 tablespoons onion flakes
2 tablespoons dried goji berries (optional)

- Preheat the oven to 400°F. Line a baking sheet with parchment paper.

- In a food processor or mixing bowl, place the almond meal, arrowroot, salt, baking powder, nutritional yeast, and chili powder. Mix well.

- Add the lemon juice, egg, coconut butter, and water and mix well. The dough should be like thick cooked oatmeal.

- Pulse or stir in the onion flakes and goji berries, if using, so they remain in large pieces. Drop balls of batter 1½ inches onto the baking sheet, in rustic, slightly irregular sizes.

- Bake for 14 to 18 minutes or until golden brown. Remove from the oven and enjoy warm.

Gluten-free	Dairy-free	Egg-free	Meat-free	Tree Nut-free	Vegan	Diabetic-friendly	Candida-friendly	High-protein	10 minutes or less
●	●		●			●	●		

SWEET POTATO ROSEMARY BISCUITS

These savory biscuits are crispy on the outside, soft and rich in the middle. Sweet potatoes give them high nutrition from beta-carotene and vitamin A, plus a bright orange color. These taste delightful with raw honey, Paleo Butter (page 45), or Paleo Cream Cheese (page 43). Freeze leftovers individually wrapped. Reheat them in an oven or a toaster oven.

YIELD: About eight biscuits • **EQUIPMENT:** A food processor is helpful but not required

1 cup almond meal
½ teaspoon unprocessed salt
¼ teaspoon baking soda
1 tablespoon ground white chia seeds (optional)
⅓ cup (75 grams) Coconut Butter (page 33); if mixing by hand,
    soften butter by placing the container in a bowl of warm water
1 large egg
½ cup (about 100 grams) raw sweet potato pulp
    (if mixing by hand, cooked and mashed)
1 teaspoon apple cider vinegar
1½ teaspoons chopped rosemary
1 tablespoon olive oil

- Preheat the oven to 350°F. Line a baking sheet with parchment paper.

- In a mixing bowl or food processor, place the almond meal, salt, baking soda, and chia seeds, if using. Mix well. Add coconut butter and mix well. To the mixture, add egg, sweet potato, vinegar, rosemary, and olive oil. Mix well. The dough will be thick like cooked oatmeal.

- Use a bit less than a ¼ cup measure to drop the batter on the baking sheet.

- Bake for 20 minutes, or until golden brown on the bottom.

Tip: If you don't have a sweet potato handy, squash or pumpkin pulp will also make tasty biscuits.

Gluten-free	Dairy-free	Egg-free	Meat-free	Tree Nut–free	Vegan	Diabetic-friendly	Candida-friendly	High-protein	10 minutes or less
●	●		●			●	●		

BACON CHILI CORNBREAD

Here is a grain-free cornbread that's just as rich, yellow, and crumbly as conventional cornbread, except it uses coconut and chia seeds. The bacon adds a rich flavor; be sure to look for bacon that's GMO- and sugar-free. I also recommend the tasty variations below: Green Chile Bacon Cornbread and Classic Cornbread or Corn Muffins. These mouthwatering breads taste even yummier with Orange Honey Butter (page 251) or Chipotle Butter (page 250).

YIELD: One 9-inch square pan cornbread, 24 mini muffins, or 10 regular muffins •
EQUIPMENT: Food processor

4 large eggs
1 tablespoon ground white chia seeds
3 tablespoons lemon juice
1 teaspoon vinegar
4 cups shredded unsweetened coconut
¾ cup almond meal
½ teaspoon unprocessed salt
½ teaspoon baking soda
1 teaspoon chili powder
¼ teaspoon pure chipotle powder
2 tablespoons nutritional yeast
½ cup Homemade Bacon Bits (page 42), or cooked, diced bacon (optional)

- Preheat the oven to 350°F. Line a 9-inch square pan with parchment paper. For muffins, grease the cups with coconut oil, and dust with coconut flour.

- In a mixing bowl whisk together the eggs, chia seeds, lemon juice, and vinegar. Mix well and set aside for a few minutes while the chia thickens.

- In a food processor place the shredded coconut. Spin it for a minute to grind the coconut. Open the machine, scrape the sides with a spatula, and spin it for another minute to grind as fine as possible. To the coconut, add almond meal, salt, baking soda, chili powder, chipotle powder, and nutritional yeast. Mix well.

- Add the wet ingredients to the dry ingredients in the processor (this begins the rising action). Mix briefly until the dough is thick like cooked oatmeal.

continues

- Pulse in the bacon so it remains in chunks and spoon the batter into the baking pan or muffin cups.

- Bake a 9-inch square pan for 30 minutes, regular muffins for 18 to 23 minutes, and mini muffins for 14 to 18 minutes, or until golden brown and a toothpick comes out clean.

VARIATIONS

Green Chile Bacon Cornbread: Follow the previous recipe. When adding the bacon pieces, pulse in a well-drained 7-ounce can of diced green chiles (mild or hot). You can also use a ½ cup of chopped roasted green chiles (Anaheim or Hatch).

Classic Cornbread or Corn Muffins: Follow the main recipe, but omit the lemon juice, spices, nutritional yeast, and bacon. Add 1 tablespoon optional sweetener, if desired.

Gluten-free	Dairy-free	Egg-free	Meat-free	Tree Nut–free	Vegan	Diabetic-friendly	Candida-friendly	High-protein	10 minutes or less
●	●					●	●		

CHIA CORN TORTILLAS

These easy, flavorful wraps are similar to Mexican tortillas or Indian chapati. They're a versatile tortilla, loaded with protein and omega-3 nutrition from chia seeds. Fill them with your favorite foods and leftovers, such as Chicken Adobo (page 229), or Spicy Chorizo (page 237). Use them in tacos, instead of bread, or any way you'd use traditional Mexican tortillas. Be aware of the size of your eggs. If they're larger than average, the dough will be runny, and if they're small the dough will be dry. I solve this problem by weighing the eggs. A large egg = 55 grams; 2 eggs = 110 grams. Freeze leftovers on a paper plate with parchment paper in between each one, in a freezer bag. That way you can pull out what you need for a super-quick breakfast.

YIELD: Seven tortillas • **EQUIPMENT:** A food processor is helpful but not required; a tortilla press or rolling pin; a digital scale is optional

6 tablespoons arrowroot flour
5 tablespoons finely ground white chia seeds
2 tablespoons shredded unsweetened coconut
2 tablespoons coconut flour
3/8 teaspoon unprocessed salt (a bit less than 1/2 teaspoon)
2 large eggs (110 grams)
2 cloves garlic, crushed
3 tablespoons coconut oil, melted but not scalding
  (place a container in a bowl of warm water)
2 tablespoons onion flakes (optional)

- In a food processor or mixing bowl, place the arrowroot, chia seeds, shredded coconut, coconut flour, and salt. Mix well—it is ideal to grind or crush these ingredients together into a powder. Then add the eggs, garlic, coconut oil, and onion flakes, if using. Mix well until the dough is quite thick, like soft clay. Wrap the dough in parchment paper or plastic wrap and allow it to rest at room temperature for at least 15 minutes. If the dough is still too wet to roll out, knead it with a bit more coconut flour.

- Roll the dough into a cylinder, and cut it into seven equal-size pieces. Roll each piece into a ball and dust with coconut flour. Place the ball in a tortilla press or roll it with a rolling pin until it is a flat, round tortilla shape. Use plastic wrap on a tortilla press. If you're rolling the dough out, roll it between two pieces of parchment paper.

continues

- Heat a nonstick pan over medium high heat. Dust your hands with a bit of coconut flour to prevent the dough from sticking to them. Gently pull the plastic or parchment away from one side of the flattened tortilla, and flip it into your floured hand. Then pull the plastic or parchment away from the other side and flip the tortilla into the heated pan.

- Cook very briefly (less than a minute) on each side. Do not overcook or it will be stiff. Adjust heat if necessary so it cooks quickly, but the oil doesn't burn. You want it to be cooked through but flexible so you can bend it around your favorite fillings. Place the finished tortillas on a plate covered with a cloth to keep them moist.

Gluten-free	Dairy-free	Egg-free	Meat-free	Tree Nut–free	Vegan	Diabetic-friendly	Candida-friendly	High-protein	10 minutes or less
●	●		●	●		●	●		

PLANTAIN TORTILLAS

These grain-free vegan tortillas share the rich flavor of plantains—which are a favorite in Africa and the Caribbean. Look for a green plantain, for its beneficial resistant starch, which is not digested like other carbs but instead it passes through the body unchanged like insoluble fiber. An aid for weight control, resistant starch increases fat burning and reduces sugar cravings. The chia seeds not only act as a binding agent, they are also a great source of omega-3s and protein. These tortillas are easy to make and tasty with Chicken Adobo (page 229), Avocado Pesto (page 252), or leftovers from last night's dinner. Freeze leftovers on a paper plate with a piece of parchment between each tortilla for up to 3 months.

YIELD: Eight tortillas • **EQUIPMENT:** A food processor; a tortilla press is optional

1 green plantain (about 240 grams), in chunks
5 tablespoons ground white chia seeds
2 tablespoons coconut flour

½ teaspoon unprocessed salt
1 clove garlic
2 tablespoons coconut oil

- In a food processor, place the plantain and process until it is liquefied. Add the remaining ingredients. Mix well. The dough will be the consistency of wet clay.

- Remove the dough from the processor and wrap in parchment paper or plastic wrap. Allow it to rest for 15 minutes at room temperature so the chia and coconut flour absorb the moisture.

- Remove the paper or plastic from the dough. Grease your hands with a bit of coconut oil or dust with coconut flour. Roll the dough into a cylinder. Cut it into seven or eight equal-size pieces. Roll each piece with your hands into a round ball. Place the ball in a tortilla press covered with plastic wrap. Or roll it with a rolling pin between two pieces of parchment paper until it is a flat round 6 to 7 inches in diameter.

- Add coconut oil to a nonstick pan and heat over medium high heat. Gently peel away the top layer of parchment paper or plastic wrap, take the tortilla in your hand, and plop it into the hot pan.

- Cook until golden brown, about 1 minute, then flip and cook the other side for an additional minute. Put finished tortillas on a plate covered with a moist towel to keep them from drying out. Enjoy!

Gluten-free	Dairy-free	Egg-free	Meat-free	Tree Nut-free	Vegan	Diabetic-friendly	Candida-friendly	High-protein	10 minutes or less
●	●	●	●	●	●	●	●		

EASY BURRITO WRAPS

Like a Southwest-style crepe, this is a flexible wrap you can fill and use for the Breakfast Burritos (page 177), Beef Fajitas with Spicy Cheese Sauce (page 228), Chicken Adobo (page 229), or even last night's leftovers. These wraps are more delicate and quicker to make than the Chia Corn Tortillas (page 73) or the Plantain Tortillas (page 75). They're a wholesome and satisfying alternative to bread; you can wrap them around most anything, secure with a toothpick, and eat with your hands. Since eggs are never a standard 55 grams, you may need to adjust the batter a wee bit. To thin, add a teaspoon more water. To thicken, add arrowroot a teaspoon at a time until it reaches easy pourable thickness. Freeze leftovers on a paper plate with parchment paper between the layers, in a freezer bag, so it's easy to pull them out when you need them.

YIELD: Three tortillas • **EQUIPMENT:** A food processor or blender is helpful but not required

2 large eggs (110 grams)
4 teaspoons ground white chia seeds
2 tablespoons filtered water
2 tablespoons arrowroot flour
¼ teaspoon unprocessed salt
2 teaspoons olive or coconut oil
2 teaspoons olive or coconut oil for cooking

- In a small blender, food processor, or small mixing bowl, place all the ingredients and mix well. The batter should be quite thin, like a crepe. Add 1 teaspoon oil to a nonstick skillet over medium high heat. Flick a few drops of water on it to see if it sizzles, and then it's ready.

- Each tortilla should have a bit less than ⅓ cup of batter. Pour it into the hot pan and tilt the pan, rotating it so the batter spreads in a round circle. It should be very thin and 7½ to 8 inches wide. Watch it cook—the edges will begin to dry out first, and then the center—about 1 minute. Gently release the edges with the corner of a spatula when they begin to pull away naturally. Then flip it over by lifting it with your fingers or a spatula. Cook briefly on the second side for about 1 minute. Don't overcook or the tortilla will be brittle. Place the finished tortillas on a plate covered with a cloth. Clean the pan with a towel and add a bit more oil. Repeat for two more tortillas.

Gluten-free	Dairy-free	Egg-free	Meat-free	Tree Nut-free	Vegan	Diabetic-friendly	Candida-friendly	High-protein	10 minutes or less
●	●		●	●		●	●		

FOCACCIA FLAT BREAD, EGG-FREE

Like a Mediterranean flat bread with a toasty onion flavor, this focaccia is one of the best-kept secrets to an easy breakfast. Quick to make and egg-free, it's a great basic bread to keep on hand for instant meals and snacks. This bread is perfect for Open-Faced Focaccia with Sausage (page 179), Chicken Adobo (page 229), leftovers, or just scrambled eggs. Freeze the bread on a paper plate with parchment paper in between the layers, placed in a freezer bag. You can defrost these in seconds, warm them in the oven, and add toppings for a quick meal.

YIELD: Eight focaccia, 6 inches in diameter • **EQUIPMENT:** A food processor is helpful but not required

1 cup filtered water
½ cup ground white chia seeds
¼ cup olive oil
1 tablespoon apple cider vinegar
2 cups almond meal
½ teaspoon baking soda
¾ teaspoon unprocessed salt

2 tablespoons onion flakes
Coconut flour for dusting

OPTIONAL TOPPINGS:
2 tablespoons olive oil
2 tablespoons sunflower seeds
2 tablespoons sesame seeds

- Preheat the oven to 400°F. Line a baking sheet with parchment paper.

- In a small bowl, stir together the water, chia seeds, olive oil, and vinegar. Allow it to sit for at least 15 minutes to thicken.

- In a mixing bowl or food processor, place the almond meal, baking soda, salt, and onion flakes. Mix well.

- Add the chia mixture and mix again. The dough will be the consistency of thick cooked oatmeal.

- Cut the dough into eight equal pieces. Roll each into a ball with your hands. Press each ball flat on a parchment paper and spread it with your fingers to 6 inches in diameter. Dust the parchment paper with coconut flour to keep from sticking. Or use a rolling pin to roll the balls between two pieces of parchment paper. Place each piece onto the baking tray.

- Rub with olive oil and sprinkle with seeds, if using, pressing them in with your hands.

- Bake for 15 to 18 minutes, until barely golden-brown on the bottom.

Gluten-free	Dairy-free	Egg-free	Meat-free	Tree Nut–free	Vegan	Diabetic-friendly	Candida-friendly	High-protein	10 minutes or less
●	●	●	●		●	●	●		

GARLIC NAAN

This easy Middle Eastern–style flatbread is grain-free, yet it is surprisingly similar to that irresistible garlic naan I used to love in Indian restaurants. This is super-quick to make in a pan, just mix the batter and cook like a pancake. It's a tasty wrap for just about everything, such as eggs, veggies, meat, or leftovers. Slather it with Avocado Pesto (page 252) or use it as a wrap for Italian Baked Eggs (page 204). The onion flakes are really tasty! Freeze with parchment paper between the layers, on a paper plate, in a freezer bag.

YIELD: Four breads, 6 to 7 inches each • **EQUIPMENT:** A food processor or small blender make it easier but are not required

2 large eggs (110 grams)
½ tablespoon coconut or olive oil
1 to 2 cloves garlic, crushed or diced
¼ teaspoon apple cider vinegar
¼ teaspoon unprocessed salt
Black pepper, to taste
¼ cup arrowroot flour
½ cup almond meal or a little bit more if needed
½ tablespoon dry herbs, such as oregano, basil, tarragon, or rosemary
1 tablespoon onion flakes (optional)
1 tablespoon coconut or olive oil for cooking

- In a food processor, small blender, or mixing bowl, place the eggs, oil, garlic, vinegar, salt, pepper, arrowroot, almond meal, herbs, and onion flakes, if using. Mix well.

- The batter should be quite liquid, like thin pancake batter. If it's too thick to pour into the pan, add a bit of water a tablespoon at a time until it is a gooey, pourable batter. If it is too liquid, add a bit of almond meal until it resembles pancake batter.

- Put ½ tablespoon oil into a nonstick skillet over medium-high heat. Test with a few drops of water to see if it sizzles, to make sure it's ready. Measure ¼ cup batter into the pan and roll the pan around like a crepe pan to spread the batter thin; or spread it with a spatula to 6 or 7 inches in diameter. Cook for about 2 minutes on each side. Place finished bread on a plate covered with a towel to keep warm. Repeat with remaining batter.

Gluten-free	Dairy-free	Egg-free	Meat-free	Tree Nut-free	Vegan	Diabetic-friendly	Candida-friendly	High-protein	10 minutes or less
●	●		●			●	●		

3

INSTANT SMOOTHIES, BEVERAGES, AND PARFAITS

"Eat food. Not too much. Mostly plants."
—Michael Pollan

How to wake up to a smoothie:

1. Get out of bed
2. Yawn
3. Place the ingredients in a blender and press start
4. Pour into a glass and drink
5. Smile

Seriously, smoothies can be your instant alternative to sugar and caffeine. Blended smoothies are the world's quickest breakfasts, an easy way to nourish your body with essential nutrients. Real food is a tonic to the whole body. It can wake you up even better than coffee.

But smoothies aren't the only easy, convenient breakfasts out there. This chapter also contains the most delectable parfaits on the planet, like Lemon Berry Parfait (page 94) and Chia Tapioca Fruit Parfait (page 93). All you need is a tall glass and a bit of fruit to make yourself an instant gourmet breakfast. And if you're missing your Caramel Macchiato or Chai Tea Latte from StarBucks, be deprived no more. You can enjoy your favorite brew and give your blood sugar a break with these Paleo-style recipes.

———

BLUEBERRY ORANGE SMOOTHIE

This morning delight will give you a healthy boost with high-antioxidant blueberries and cranberries, with honey and a hint of ginger.

YIELD: Serves one • **EQUIPMENT:** Any blender or food processor

¾ cup filtered water, coconut milk (page 35), almond milk, or hemp milk (page 36)
¾ cup blueberries
¼ cup whole cranberries
½ orange
1 teaspoon bee pollen (optional)
1 scoop of your favorite protein powder
1-inch piece fresh ginger root, diced
1 teaspoon sweetener (optional); I suggest raw honey or
    ½ tablespoon zero-carb sweetener (see page 18 for options)

• Blend all ingredients until liquefied. Pour into a tall glass and enjoy immediately.

Gluten-free	Dairy-free	Egg-free	Meat-free	Tree Nut–free	Vegan	Diabetic-friendly	Candida-friendly	High-protein	10 minutes or less
●	●	●	●	●	●	●	●	●	●

What Makes a Great Smoothie, and What Doesn't?

1. Use whole fresh fruit and veggies including the stems and seeds and skins, when appropriate. Whole fresh fruits and vegetables are rich in phytochemicals that nourish our body's organs and endocrine system. These phytochemicals are often hidden in the cellulose fibers of seeds, stems, skins, and rinds of fruits and vegetables. Many of us eat the best foods, but we throw away the most nutritious parts. When we eat fruits and veggies in their whole form we are getting pulp and fiber to help slow down the absorption of natural sugars in these foods—and this helps to balance metabolism. Even fruit juices, a favorite breakfast beverage that many would consider "healthy," are high in fructose sugar, and low in fiber. As processed extractions from fruit, juices have no place in a low-carb Paleo diet. It's far better to go for the real thing—the whole unprocessed fruit.

2. Get a great blender. A super-blender such as the Blendtec or Vitamix can micronize the food to release the phytochemicals. See Tools (page 25). The best blenders literally break through the cell walls of your food, which makes it easier for your body to digest. More important, they can also increase the amount of nutrients that flow into your bloodstream. This is especially important for athletes, moms, anyone with a stressful job, or those suffering from digestive disorders. You can break out or "micronize" phytochemicals from the seeds, stems, skins, and rinds to maximize nutrient absorption.

3. Eat Low-Sugar Fruits
   - The best Paleo fruits are the lowest in natural fructose sugar, such as blueberries, raspberries, Granny Smith apples, lemons, limes, cranberries, elderberries, and gooseberries.
   - Eat limited quantities of medium-sweet fruit, such as papaya, grapefruit, kiwi, strawberries, tangerine, and kumquat.
   - Avoid high-sugar fruits and juices, such as mango, pineapple, and orange. Stay away from high-sugar dried fruits, such as dates, raisins, figs, apricots, and prunes, to give your blood sugar a break. Instead, try using cinnamon, spices, and chopped nuts to jazz up your breakfast.

4. Drink up! Smoothies begin oxidizing immediately unless stored in a completely air-free container, so to get the most out of your drinks, you should consume smoothies immediately.

BERRY GRAPEFRUIT SMOOTHIE WITH GREENS

With red berries, grapefruit, greens, and pumpkin seeds, this smoothie is vitalizing and refreshing.

YIELD: Serves one • **EQUIPMENT:** Any blender or food processor

½ cup filtered water or coconut water
1 cup tart red berries, such as raspberries and strawberries
½ grapefruit
½-inch piece ginger root, diced
1 teaspoon bee pollen (optional)
1 scoop of your favorite protein powder
A handful baby spinach or your favorite greens
1 tablespoon pumpkin seeds (optional)
Sweetener is optional, 0 to 1 teaspoon (see options on page 18)

• Blend all ingredients until liquefied. Pour into a tall glass and enjoy immediately.

Gluten-free	Dairy-free	Egg-free	Meat-free	Tree Nut–free	Vegan	Diabetic-friendly	Candida-friendly	High-protein	10 minutes or less
●	●	●	●	●	●	●	●	●	●

CHOCOLATE ALMOND PICK-ME-UP

This smoothie is an energy powerhouse of strawberries, cacao, almond butter vanilla, cinnamon, and protein.

YIELD: Serves one • **EQUIPMENT:** Any blender or food processor

¾ cup filtered water, coconut milk (page 35),
    almond milk, or hemp milk (page 36)
2 tablespoons pure cacao powder, or carob powder, or 1 of each
1 to 2 handfuls strawberries
¼ cup almond butter (page 38)
2 to 3 teaspoons raw honey, or 1 tablespoon zero-carb sweetener
    (see page 18 for options), sweeten to taste
1 tablespoon maca powder
1 scoop of your favorite protein powder
½ teaspoon ground cinnamon
1 teaspoon vanilla
¼ beet, in chunks
¼ teaspoon instant decaf coffee crystals (optional) for mocha flavor

• Blend all ingredients until liquefied. Pour into a tall glass and enjoy immediately.

Gluten-free	Dairy-free	Egg-free	Meat-free	Tree Nut–free	Vegan	Diabetic-friendly	Candida-friendly	High-protein	10 minutes or less
●	●	●	●					●	●

CRAN-APPLE SPICE SMOOTHIE

This invigorating blend of cranberries, apple, cinnamon, spices, vanilla, and protein power is a taste of autumn, any time of the year.

YIELD: Serves one • **EQUIPMENT:** Any blender or food processor

¾ cup filtered water, coconut milk (page 35), almond milk, or hemp milk (page 36)
1 tart apple, like Granny Smith, Fuji, or Pink Lady
2 handfuls frozen unsweetened cranberries
1 teaspoon ground cinnamon
A pinch of cardamom
A pinch of cloves
A dash of vanilla
1 teaspoon bee pollen (optional)
1-inch piece fresh ginger root, diced
1 large scoop protein power

• Blend all ingredients until liquefied. Pour into a tall glass and enjoy immediately.

Gluten-free	Dairy-free	Egg-free	Meat-free	Tree Nut–free	Vegan	Diabetic-friendly	Candida-friendly	High-protein	10 minutes or less
●	●	●	●	●	●	●	●	●	●

HIGH-PROTEIN KEFIR BERRY SMOOTHIE

A creamy shake with high-antioxidant berries and goat kefir, inspired by the healing discoveries of Dr. Johanna Budwig, German physician and seven-time Nobel Prize nominee. Basically a fermented kefir drink with flax oil and fruit, it is loaded with protein, omega-3 fatty acids, and flavor.

YIELD: Serves one • **EQUIPMENT:** Any blender or food processor

½ cup goat kefir or coconut kefir
½ cup filtered water, coconut milk (page 35), almond milk, or hemp milk (page 36)
2 tablespoons flax oil
½ cup low-sugar berries, such as raspberries, blueberries,
    gooseberries, elderberries, and/or cranberries. They should
    be unsweetened, fresh or frozen.
½ orange, peeled
½ teaspoon vanilla
1 scoop of your favorite protein powder
1 teaspoon bee pollen (optional)
2 teaspoons maca powder
Sweetener is optional, 1 to 2 tablespoons (see options on page 18)

• Blend all ingredients until liquefied. Pour into a tall glass and enjoy immediately.

Gluten-free	Dairy-free	Egg-free	Meat-free	Tree Nut–free	Vegan	Diabetic-friendly	Candida-friendly	High-protein	10 minutes or less
●		●	●	●		●		●	●

PAPAYA BERRY SMOOTHIE

A tropical smoothie, red-orange in color, with sweet papaya and nuances of orange. The succulent papaya fruit is a favorite for its digestive, medicinal, and nutritional benefits. It's also relatively low in sugar, a great boon for Paleo dieters. Look for organic papaya, as conventional varieties are most likely genetically modified.

YIELD: Serves one • **EQUIPMENT:** Any blender or food processor

½ cup unsweetened coconut milk (page 35), almond milk, or hemp milk (page 36), or filtered water
1 small papaya, peeled, seeded, and cubed
1 handful strawberries or raspberries
¼ teaspoon ground cinnamon
Zest of one-half orange
½ orange, peeled and seeded
1 scoop of your favorite protein powder

• Blend all ingredients until liquefied. Pour into a tall glass and enjoy immediately.

Gluten-free	Dairy-free	Egg-free	Meat-free	Tree Nut-free	Vegan	Diabetic-friendly	Candida-friendly	High-protein	10 minutes or less
●	●	●	●	●	●	●	●	●	●

PEACHES AND GREENS SMOOTHIE

This vibrant, creamy blend of peaches, berries, and greens makes an enjoyable alternative to caffeine. The delicate pungent flavor comes from ginger, a potent natural elixir for digestion, sinus health, and energy vitality.

YIELD: Serves one • **EQUIPMENT:** Any blender or food processor

½ cup unsweetened coconut milk (page 35), almond milk,
   hemp milk (page 36), or filtered water
1 whole peach or nectarine, sliced, or frozen equivalent
1 handful berries, such as raspberries or strawberries
1 teaspoon bee pollen (optional)
1 scoop of your favorite green powder
1 scoop your favorite protein powder
1 handful fresh greens, such as baby spinach, fennel tops, or chard
1 slice lemon without the peel
½-inch piece fresh ginger root, peeled and diced
¼ teaspoon ground cinnamon

• Blend all ingredients until liquefied. Pour into a tall glass and enjoy immediately.

Gluten-free	Dairy-free	Egg-free	Meat-free	Tree Nut–free	Vegan	Diabetic-friendly	Candida-friendly	High-protein	10 minutes or less
●	●	●	●	●	●	●	●	●	●

STRAWBERRY BEET SMOOTHIE

A wake-me-up smoothie in a deep pink color from—you guessed it—beets! These often-forgotten veggies boost morning vitality and help regulate the immune system. They're a potent source of iron and guard against cancer. Strawberries add a sweet flavor and antioxidant boost.

YIELD: Serves one • **EQUIPMENT:** Any blender or food processor

¾ cup filtered water or coconut water
A large handful strawberries
½ small beet, in chunks
½ tart apple, such as Fuji, Pink Lady, Granny Smith, or 4 crab-apples
1 scoop of your favorite protein powder
½-inch piece fresh ginger root
2 tablespoons hemp nuts
Zest of one-half orange (optional)

• Blend all ingredients until liquefied. Pour into a tall glass and enjoy immediately.

Gluten-free	Dairy-free	Egg-free	Meat-free	Tree Nut-free	Vegan	Diabetic-friendly	Candida-friendly	High-protein	10 minutes or less
●	●	●	●	●	●	●	●	●	●

SUNRISE GREEN SMOOTHIE

This is my personal favorite green smoothie, which you can vary in so many ways. Choose delicate baby spinach leaves, mellow kale, or slightly tart beet tops. Select your berries and type of apple so that every morning's recipe is unique and a tantalizing surprise.

YIELD: Serves one • **EQUIPMENT:** Any blender or food processor

1 cup filtered water
4 leaves raw kale, beet tops, or handful spinach leaves
1 tart apple, such as Granny Smith, Fuji, or Pink Lady
½ medium carrot, in chunks
½-inch piece fresh ginger root, peeled and chopped
½ lemon or lime, peeled and seeded
Sweetener is optional, 0 to 1 tablespoon (see options on page 18)
½ cup tart berries (blueberries, raspberries, blackberries, açai, gooseberries, or elderberries)
1 scoop of your favorite protein powder
3 tablespoons of your favorite green powder
1 dropper-full of ChlorOxygen Alcohol-Free Chlorophyll by Herbs Etc.
¼ cup roasted almond butter or sunflower butter (page 38)

• Blend all ingredients until liquefied. Pour into a tall glass and enjoy immediately.

Gluten-free	Dairy-free	Egg-free	Meat-free	Tree Nut–free	Vegan	Diabetic-friendly	Candida-friendly	High-protein	10 minutes or less
●	●	●	●		●	●	●	●	●

FRUIT WITH COCONUT CREAM TOPPING

This is one of the quickest and tastiest breakfasts you can enjoy in minutes. Slice up your favorite fruit and serve with Coconut Cream Topping (page 249).

YIELD: Serves one

1 recipe Coconut Cream Topping (page 249)

Here are some low-sugar fruit combination ideas:

Berries and grapefruit

Apples and pears with cinnamon

Mixed berries, such as blueberries, raspberries, and /or elderberries

Blueberries, kumquat, kiwi

Papaya and strawberries, sprinkled and tossed with lime juice

Gluten-free	Dairy-free	Egg-free	Meat-free	Tree Nut-free	Vegan	Diabetic-friendly	Candida-friendly	High-protein	10 minutes or less
●	●	●	●	●	●	●	●		●

BLUE MOUSSE

Once in a blue mousse, you discover something so easy and fabulicious that it jump-starts your day in 2 minutes! This creamy blueberry mousse has a smooth texture and yummy flavor for vital health. It's instant—just blend and eat immediately. The thick texture comes from natural pectin in blueberries and creamy avocado. Blueberries are loaded with healthy anthocyanins, powerful antioxidants that neutralize free radicals in the body.

YIELD: Serves two • **EQUIPMENT:** Any blender

¾ cup unsweetened coconut milk (page 35) or almond milk (page 36)
1½ tablespoons lemon juice
1½ cups fresh blueberries, or 1 cup if frozen
2 tablespoons coconut oil (optional)
2 to 6 tablespoons sweetener, to taste (see options on page 18)
2 teaspoons vanilla
A pinch of unprocessed salt
1 ripe avocado, peeled and pitted

- In any blender, place milk, lemon juice, blueberries, coconut oil, if using, sweetener, vanilla, and salt. Blend until smooth and creamy.

- Add the avocado last and blend well.

- Pour into 2 serving glasses. Enjoy immediately for the most beautiful blue color. The color will fade slightly over time, but it will still be delicious!

Gluten-free	Dairy-free	Egg-free	Meat-free	Tree Nut-free	Vegan	Diabetic-friendly	Candida-friendly	High-protein	10 minutes or less
●	●	●	●	●	●	●	●		●

RASPBERRY CHEESECAKE PARFAIT

How about a heavenly cheesecake mousse layered with pecans and raspberries? It's a delightful way to start the day. Raspberries are high in the antioxidant ellagic acid, a known anticarcinogen. Plus raspberries are relatively low in fructose sugars, to help keep your blood sugar levels stable through the day. This easy cheesecake mousse is 100 percent dairy-free, made with coconut butter and lemon.

YIELD: Serves one • **EQUIPMENT:** A small blender, immersion blender, or food processor

¾ cup unsweetened coconut milk (page 35)
2 tablespoons lemon juice
⅓ cup (75 grams) Coconut Butter (page 33), softened
  (place the container in a bowl of warm water)
1 teaspoon vanilla
⅛ teaspoon unprocessed salt
About 2 tablespoons sweetener to taste (see options on page 18)
¼ cup pecans, soaked and toasted if possible (page 40)
½ cup raspberries, fresh or frozen

- Blend all ingredients except the pecans and raspberries in a food processor, a high-speed blender with a small container, or an immersion blender.

- Layer the mousse in a glass with pecans and fresh raspberries.

Gluten-free	Dairy-free	Egg-free	Meat-free	Tree Nut-free	Vegan	Diabetic-friendly	Candida-friendly	High-protein	10 minutes or less
●	●	●	●		●	●	●		●

CHIA TAPIOCA FRUIT PARFAIT

The word "chia" is a Mayan word meaning strength. Chia seeds are a perfectly balanced blend of protein, omega-3 fatty acids, and fiber—truly a superfood. One of the simplest breakfasts you can make, this parfait tastes heavenly with any fruit. You can use white or black chia seeds; white seeds make it look like old-fashioned tapioca.

YIELD: Serves one

3 tablespoons chia seeds, white or black
¾ cup unsweetened coconut milk (page 35) or almond milk (page 36)
1 teaspoon vanilla
A sprinkle of ground cinnamon
Sweetener is optional, 0 to 2 teaspoons (see options on page 18)
¾ cup low-sugar colorful fruit, such as raspberries, blueberries, kiwi, kumquat, etc.

- In a cereal bowl, stir together chia seeds, milk, vanilla, cinnamon, and optional sweetener. Let it sit for 15 minutes or refrigerate overnight, and the chia seeds will expand, soften, and absorb the liquid.

- Layer chia tapioca in a tall glass with your favorite fruit.

Gluten-free	Dairy-free	Egg-free	Meat-free	Tree Nut–free	Vegan	Diabetic-friendly	Candida-friendly	High-protein	10 minutes or less
●	●	●	●	●	●	●	●		●

LEMON BERRY PARFAIT

A refreshing lemon mousse layered with berries—your wholesome fruit breakfast is ready in 5 minutes. Powerful antioxidants in berries such as anthocyanins, quercetin, and vitamin C help to reduce inflammation and fight oxidative stress caused by free radicals. Almonds are an important source of protein and fiber, while being naturally low in sugar.

YIELD: Serves one • **EQUIPMENT:** Food processor, high-speed blender with small jar, or immersion blender with cup

½ cup unsweetened coconut milk (page 35),
  or a bit more if needed to blend
½ cup (113 grams) Coconut Butter (page 33), softened
  (place the container in a bowl of warm water)
Zest of 1 lemon
2 tablespoons lemon juice
Zest of 1 orange
A dash of vanilla
About 3 tablespoons sweetener to taste (see options on page 18)
¾ cup tart berries, such as blueberries, raspberries,
  strawberries, gooseberries
¼ cup almonds, soaked and toasted if possible (page 40)

- Blend all ingredients except the berries and almonds in a food processor, high-speed blender with a small jar, or an immersion blender with a cup.

- Layer the lemon mousse in a tall glass with toasted almonds and tart berries.

Gluten-free	Dairy-free	Egg-free	Meat-free	Tree Nut–free	Vegan	Diabetic-friendly	Candida-friendly	High-protein	10 minutes or less
●	●	●	●		●	●	●		●

PUMPKIN BANANA NUT PARFAIT

A seasonal favorite, pumpkin deserves to play a more important role in your diet all year-round. Pumpkins are loaded with vitamin A, to keep your eyes sharp. They're also a rich source of healthy fiber and antioxidants. Blend this easy pumpkin mousse with cinnamon and spices, then layer yourself a parfait with banana and cacao nibs.

YIELD: Serves one • **EQUIPMENT NEEDED:** None, but a small blender is helpful

1 cup cooked pumpkin pulp, butternut squash, or sweet potato
3 to 4 tablespoons unsweetened coconut milk (page 35) or almond milk (page 36)
½ teaspoon pumpkin pie spice
A splash of vanilla
A pinch of unprocessed salt
Sweetener is optional, 0 to 2 tablespoons, part brown sweetener
    (see options on page 18)
½ banana, sliced
¼ cup walnuts, soaked and toasted if possible (page 40)
A handful of unsweetened cacao nibs (optional)

- Blend or mash the pumpkin by hand, or in a food processor, a high-speed blender with a small container, or an immersion blender with a cup. Add milk, spice, vanilla, salt, and sweetener, if using. Mix well.

- Layer the pumpkin mousse in a tall glass with banana slices, toasted nuts, and unsweetened cacao nibs.

Gluten-free	Dairy-free	Egg-free	Meat-free	Tree Nut–free	Vegan	Diabetic-friendly	Candida-friendly	High-protein	10 minutes or less
●	●	●	●		●	●	●		●

BLUEBERRY HEMP PARFAIT

Here's a creamy and satisfying parfait with blueberries, kiwi, and hemp mousse. Hemp nuts are amazing—a true superfood that contains the ideal balance of amino acids and fatty acids necessary for human health. No other single plant has the essential amino acids in such an easily digestible form. So easy to make, just mix, layer, and enjoy.

YIELD: Serves one • **EQUIPMENT NEEDED:** A food processor or high-speed blender with small container

¾ cup hemp nuts
1 teaspoon vanilla
2 teaspoons lemon juice
4 to 5 tablespoons unsweetened coconut milk (page 35)
Sweetener is optional, 0 to 2 tablespoons (see options on page 18)
½ cup blueberries, fresh or frozen
1 kiwi fruit

- Process the hemp nuts for several minutes until they are completely liquefied into a thick cream. This will be quickest in a super-blender; it takes a bit longer in a food processor. Open the container, scrape the sides, and process again until smooth. Then add vanilla and lemon juice. Pour in the coconut milk slowly until it reaches your desired texture. Sweeten to taste.

- Layer hemp mousse in a tall glass with blueberries and kiwi slices.

Gluten-free	Dairy-free	Egg-free	Meat-free	Tree Nut-free	Vegan	Diabetic-friendly	Candida-friendly	High-protein	10 minutes or less
●	●	●	●	●	●	●	●	●	●

VANILLA CREAM PARFAIT WITH STRAWBERRIES AND PUMPKIN SEEDS

This tempting cashew cream pudding looks like whipped cream and tastes delightful with fruit. Cashews are high in iron, phosphorus, selenium, magnesium, and zinc. An excellent source of anticancer flavanols, cashews have a lower fat content than most other nuts. Easy to make, just blend the pudding and layer in a glass with strawberries and pumpkin seeds.

YIELD: Serves one • **EQUIPMENT NEEDED:** A food processor or high-speed blender with small jar

1 cup raw cashews soaked 1 to 6 hours
½ cup (or more if necessary) unsweetened coconut milk (page 35), almond milk (page 36), or filtered water
½ teaspoon vanilla
A pinch of unprocessed salt
Sweetener is optional, 0 to 2 teaspoons (see options on page 18)
½ cup sliced strawberries
A handful of pumpkin seeds, soaked and toasted if possible (page 40)

- In a food processor or high-speed blender with a small jar, place cashews, milk, vanilla, salt, and sweetener, if using. Mix to a thick and creamy texture. This will be quicker in a high-speed blender and will take a minute or two in a food processor. Add more liquid slowly if necessary until desired thickness is reached.

- In a tall glass, layer the cashew cream with strawberries and pumpkin seeds.

Gluten-free	Dairy-free	Egg-free	Meat-free	Tree Nut–free	Vegan	Diabetic-friendly	Candida-friendly	High-protein	10 minutes or less
●	●	●	●		●	●			●

CAPPUCCINO

If you secretly desire a rich Italian coffee, be deprived no more. Quick to make and 100 percent caffeine-free, this Paleo brew uses steamed coconut milk and tastes almost like the real thing. Roasted chicory root has a rich, satisfying flavor while being high in antioxidants that support healthy liver function. Dandelion is most often thought of as a weed. However dandelion root "tea" has been used in traditional Chinese and Native American medicine for centuries. Even Dr. Oz recommends it in his 48-hour liver cleanse. Personally, I enjoy the rich, satisfying flavor of my Paleo Joe. For chicory and dandelion granules, see Resources (page 271).

YIELD: Serves two • **EQUIPMENT:** A French press is helpful but not necessary

2 tablespoons roasted chicory root granules

2 tablespoons roasted dandelion root granules

4 cups boiling filtered water

Sweetener is optional, 0 to 2 tablespoons (see options on page 18)

½ cup unsweetened full-fat coconut milk (page 13), gently heated on the stove

Ground cinnamon to sprinkle

- Put the chicory and dandelion granules into a French press (or saucepan). Fill it with boiling water and allow the brew to steep for 2 minutes.

- Press the plunger (or strain). Pour the coffee into two large coffee mugs.

- To froth the milk, heat it briefly in a saucepan. Whisk it with a miniature whisk, immersion blender, or, even better, an electric milk frother until you see bubbles on the surface (see Resources, page 273). Pour it over the coffee in your mugs. Sprinkle with cinnamon. Stir in sweetener to taste.

VARIATIONS:
Caffè Latte
Follow the recipe above, except use 1 cup unsweetened coconut milk (page 35).

Mochaccino
Follow the Cappuccino recipe above, adding to the French press:
    1 tablespoon pure cacao powder
    3 to 4 tablespoons sweetener to taste (see options on page 18)
    Sprinkle a pinch of cacao powder on top

Gluten-free	Dairy-free	Egg-free	Meat-free	Tree Nut-free	Vegan	Diabetic-friendly	Candida-friendly	High-protein	10 minutes or less
●	●	●	●	●	●	●	●		●

CHAI TEA

Flavorful chai has been a traditional breakfast in Asia for centuries. I use Tulsi tea, also called Holy Basil tea, because its flavor mimics traditional tea, yet it is caffeine-free. Tulsi is considered one of the most important herbs in ayurveda, used for its ability to balance hormones and fight stress. However any dark caffeine-free tea will work. Tantalizing spices such as ginger, cardamom, and cinnamon aid digestion, improve circulation, and boost the immune system.

YIELD: Two 16-ounce cups

2 cups filtered water
2 to 4 tea bags Tulsi tea, or the equivalent loose tea
2 cups unsweetened coconut milk (page 35)
    or almond milk (page 36)
2 to 4 tablespoons sweetener to taste (see options on page 18)
1 teaspoon vanilla
A pinch of black pepper
2 teaspoons ground cinnamon
1 to 2 teaspoons ground cardamom
¼ teaspoon ground cloves
¼ teaspoon ground ginger, or 1-inch piece fresh ginger,
    peeled and sliced thinly
¼ teaspoon ground anise, or 2 pieces of star anise (optional)

- In a small saucepan, boil the filtered water. Add the tea bags, remove the water from the heat, and allow the tea to steep for 3 minutes.

- Remove the tea bags. Add milk, sweetener, vanilla, pepper, cinnamon, cardamom, cloves, ginger, and anise, if using. Stir and heat to boiling but do not boil. Remove from the heat, cover, and let steep for 3 minutes. Enjoy!

Gluten-free	Dairy-free	Egg-free	Meat-free	Tree Nut-free	Vegan	Diabetic-friendly	Candida-friendly	High-protein	10 minutes or less
●	●	●	●	●	●	●	●		●

4

GRAIN-FREE CEREALS

"Going grain free and sugar free could be
the #1 best thing you ever do for your health."
—Mark Sisson, Primal Fitness

If you've ever wondered why you would ever want to make your own grain-free cereal when there are so many delicious store brands, here's a good answer (but it's not a pretty one). All packaged cereals are made with heavy processing, even the organic ones. Cereal grains are liquefied, heated to high temperatures, and then pressured into various shapes, puffs, and flakes. These shapes are then sprayed with vegetable oil and sugar to seal the grains and give them an irresistible crunchiness—forever. Unfortunately, this processing alters the structure of the cereal grain, leaving a mixture that is tasty, nutritionally empty, and toxic. The result is that never-ending aisle of boxed cereals in every grocery, including the healthy ones. Clearly, it's time to think outside the cereal box.

Making your own breakfast cereal is quick and the only healthy way to go. The first step is to know what's a grain, and what's not. Well, grains are just cultivated grasses. The most common ones are wheat, rye, barley, rice, oats, and corn.

Well then, what's in grain-free breakfast cereal? Anything you can hunt and gather! These recipes are made of pure unprocessed, nutrient-dense nuts and seeds. They're loaded with protein, phytochemicals, antioxidants, fiber, and healthy fats. Even better, they're much lower in carbs and sugars than their processed counterparts. These recipes show you how to make your own breakfast cereals using almonds, walnuts, pecans, cashews, hazelnuts, Brazil nuts, pumpkin seeds, sunflower seeds, sesame seeds, buckwheat, coconut, chia, hemp, and flax. These are quick to make and truly flavorful, such as Coconut Flax Cereal with Berries (page 107) or Cream of Hemp with Apple and Cinnamon (page 106). To jump-start your day, top off the cereal bowl with nutrient-dense High-Protein Coconut Milk (page 35) or High-Protein Nut Milk (page 37).

You'll also find recipes for granola here—the true embodiments of a wholesome high-fiber breakfast cereal that's deliciously crunchy and healthy. Once you've tasted the full-bodied, real-food flavor of homemade Apple Cinnamon Granola (page 103) or Cocoa-Nutty Granola (page 104), you'll never go back to the store-bought granolas that are loaded with sugar, sweeteners, and have been stored so long the grains are stale. The grain-free recipes in this book are designed to be easy and to preserve the nutrients and flavors in real food. They're intended to support your health and well-being on a deep, cellular level.

APPLE CINNAMON GRANOLA

Granola is a great staple to keep on hand for a quick breakfast. This easy recipe is made with nuts, coconut, whole apple, and sweet-smelling spices. It's way better than store-bought granola because it is fresh and free of grains, sugars, and preservatives. Enjoy it with High-Protein Coconut Milk (page 35) or High-Protein Nut Milk (page 37) and fruit on top. Refrigerate in a glass jar for two weeks or in baggies in the freezer up to three months.

YIELD: 3 cups granola • **EQUIPMENT:** A food processor is helpful but not required

2½ cups mixed raw, unsalted nuts and seeds, such as almonds, walnuts, pecans, cashews, hazelnuts, Brazil nuts, pumpkin seeds, sunflower seeds, sesame seeds, soaked if possible (page 40), and coarsely chopped (chop by hand, or pulse in a food processor)

½ cup shredded unsweetened coconut

SYRUP:

⅓ cup coconut oil, melted (place the jar in a bowl of lukewarm water)

2 teaspoons vanilla

¼ teaspoon unprocessed salt

Sweetener is optional, 0 to 3 tablespoons (See options on page 18. I especially like brown sweetener in this recipe.)

1 Granny Smith apple, unpeeled, cored, cut in chunks (see directions if you are working without a food processor)

2 tablespoons ground cinnamon

¼ teaspoon ground ginger

¼ teaspoon ground cloves (optional)

¼ teaspoon grated nutmeg (optional)

Zest of one orange (optional)

- Preheat the oven to 300°F. Cover a 9 x 13-inch pan with parchment paper.

- Put the nuts in a large mixing bowl and add the shredded coconut.

- For the syrup, in a food processor or mixing bowl place the melted oil, vanilla, salt, sweetener, apple, cinnamon, ginger, cloves, nutmeg, and orange zest, if using. Process until the apple is liquefied. If you're working by hand or with a hand mixer, grate or chop the apple very finely before adding it to the wet ingredients. Add the syrup to the nuts and mix well.

- Pour the mixture into the prepared baking pan. Bake for 45 to 50 minutes, or until golden brown. Open the oven and stir every 10 minutes. (Granola burns easily, so keep an eye on it. I set two timers—one every 10 minutes to remind me to stir, and one for 45 minutes.) Remove from the oven. It will become crispy as it cools. Allow it to cool completely before storing.

Gluten-free	Dairy-free	Egg-free	Meat-free	Tree Nut–free	Vegan	Diabetic-friendly	Candida-friendly	High-protein	10 minutes or less
●	●	●	●		●	●	●		

COCOA-NUTTY GRANOLA

This crispy, toasted chocolate granola tastes so scrumptious, you'll never guess it's loaded with healthy nutrition. High protein almond meal, fresh carrot, and nuts make it a powerhouse of vitamins and minerals not found in store-bought granola. Pure cacao adds a tiny dose of tryptophan and phenethylamine for a pleasant lift as you start your day. Serve with your favorite High-Protein Nut Milk (page 37) and fruit on top. Keep the granola in a glass jar for several weeks or put it in baggies in the freezer for longer.

YIELD: 5 cups granola

½ cup coconut oil

½ cup raw honey (or ⅔ cup Just Like Sugar Table Top or Brown mixed with 3 tablespoons boiling water)

1½ teaspoons unprocessed salt

1 tablespoon vanilla

¼ teaspoon maple flavor (optional)

2 cups nuts and seeds, such as walnuts, almonds, pecans, hazelnuts, Brazil nuts, macadamia nuts, sunflower seeds, and/or pumpkin seeds, coarsely chopped. Presoak and crisp them if possible (page 40).

3 tablespoons pure cacao powder

1 tablespoon ground cinnamon

1 carrot, coarsely shredded, or a small beet

1 cup shredded unsweetened coconut

1 cup almond meal

- Preheat the oven to 300°F. Line a 9 x 13-inch pan with parchment paper.

- In a small saucepan over low heat, stir together the coconut oil, honey, salt, vanilla, and maple, if using. There's no need to cook it, just heat briefly to melt together, stirring until smooth. Remove from the heat.

- Put the nuts in a large mixing bowl. Add the cacao, cinnamon, carrot, coconut, and almond meal. Stir gently. Pour the liquid mixture over the dry ingredients and stir with a spatula until well mixed.

- Pour the granola into the baking pan. Bake for 45 to 50 minutes, stirring briefly with an oven-safe spatula every 10 minutes. (Granola burns easily, so keep an eye on it. I set two timers—one every 10 minutes, and one for 45 minutes.) This will get crispy after you remove it from the oven. Allow to cool completely before storing.

Gluten-free	Dairy-free	Egg-free	Meat-free	Tree Nut-free	Vegan	Diabetic-friendly	Candida-friendly	High-protein	10 minutes or less
●	●	●	●						

HIGH-PROTEIN CHIA-CRUNCH GRANOLA

Loaded with protein and high nutrition in nuts, pumpkin seeds, and chia seeds, this granola is bursting with the flavor of freshly toasted nuts and honey. Instead of oats, which is considered a glutinous Neolithic grain (not Paleo), this granola uses buckwheat, a seed related to rhubarb. Buckwheat is high in protein, phytochemicals, antioxidants, and fiber. Sometimes called kasha or groats, it is best soaked 6 to 8 hours before you use it. This is very tasty with cinnamon flavored Homemade Nut Milk (page 37). Keep granola in a glass jar for several weeks or put it in baggies in the freezer for longer.

YIELD: 5 cups granola

¾ cup buckwheat groats (see directions)

½ cup coconut oil

½ cup raw honey (or ⅔ cup Just Like Sugar Table Top or Brown, mixed with 3 tablespoons boiling water)

¾ teaspoon unprocessed salt

2 teaspoons vanilla

¼ teaspoon maple flavor (optional)

2½ cups nuts, such as almonds, walnuts, pecans, Brazil nuts, pumpkin seeds, sunflower seeds, etc., soaked and crisped if possible (page 40)

3 tablespoons whole chia seeds, white or black

1 teaspoon ground cinnamon

3 tablespoons of your favorite protein powder

- Soak the buckwheat groats overnight in filtered water at room temperature. Rinse and drain well.

- Preheat the oven to 300°F. Line a 9 x 13-inch pan with parchment paper.

- In a small pan over low heat, stir together the coconut oil, honey, salt, vanilla, and maple, if using. Heat very briefly, stirring until smooth, and remove from the heat.

- Chop the nuts coarsely by hand or in a food processor and place them in a large mixing bowl. Add the chia seeds, cinnamon, protein powder, and buckwheat. Stir gently. Pour the liquid honey mixture over the dry ingredients and stir with a spatula until well mixed.

- Pour the mixture into the prepared baking pan. Bake for 45 to 50 minutes, stirring with an oven-safe spatula every 10 minutes. Granola burns easily, so keep an eye on it. (I set two timers—one every 10 minutes and one for 45 minutes.) When the 50 minutes are up, the granola may seem soggy; do not worry, it crisps as it cools. Remove from the oven. Allow to cool completely before storing.

Gluten-free	Dairy-free	Egg-free	Meat-free	Tree Nut-free	Vegan	Diabetic-friendly	Candida-friendly	High-protein	10 minutes or less
●	●	●	●					●	

CREAM OF HEMP WITH APPLE AND CINNAMON

It was a cold blustery morning, and I woke up hungry. My body said hot cream of wheat, but my mind said no—it has to be Paleo, gluten- and grain-free. There were two Granny Smiths sitting on the counter, and, well, 2 minutes later I was eating a warm bowl of cream of hemp. This tasty "cereal" is loaded with protein and high omega-3 nutrition. Flaxseeds should always be used immediately after grinding—a hand-held grinder works well. If you have a super-blender such as the Vitamix or Blendtec, it's even quicker to add whole flaxseeds and let the machine grind them.

YIELD: Serves one • **EQUIPMENT:** Any blender or food processor

¾ cup hot water
2 Granny Smith apples, cored, cut in chunks with the peel
1 teaspoon ground cinnamon
1 scoop of your favorite protein powder
¼ cup flaxseeds, freshly ground
Sweetener is optional, 0 to 3 tablespoons brown sweetener
   (see options on page 18)
⅛ teaspoon maple flavor
½ cup hemp nuts

- In a blender or food processor, place the water, apples, cinnamon, protein powder, ground flaxseeds, sweetener, and maple flavor. Process until smooth and the apples are liquefied.

- Adjust sweetener, if using. Add hemp nuts last and mix briefly so they're still crunchy and not mush.

- Pour into a cereal bowl and eat.

Gluten-free	Dairy-free	Egg-free	Meat-free	Tree Nut–free	Vegan	Diabetic-friendly	Candida-friendly	High-protein	10 minutes or less
●	●	●	●	●	●	●	●	●	●

COCONUT FLAX CEREAL WITH BERRIES

If Grok could tell us his ideal breakfast, this would be it! (Grok is the mythical primal strong-man whose diet we'd like to mimic.) Quick to make, this crunchy breakfast has the warm, full-bodied flavor of coconut and toasted nuts. Freshly ground flax seeds add omega-3 fatty acids, lignans, and fiber. Flaxseeds are delicate: Preground flax oxidizes, or spoils, quickly. Unground, the seed's impermeable coating may pass right through your digestion without releasing any of the benefits. The best way to eat flaxseed is to grind well and consume it immediately. This tastes heavenly with cinnamon-flavored High-Protein Coconut Milk (page 35), or Homemade Nut Milk (page 36).

YIELD: Serves one • **EQUIPMENT:** A hand-held grinder or super-blender such as Vitamix or Blendtec

1 cup hot unsweetened coconut milk (page 35),
    or any nut milk (page 36)
¼ cup freshly ground flaxseeds
¼ cup unsweetened shredded coconut
¼ cup chopped nuts, such as pumpkin seeds, walnuts, pecans,
    almonds, or sunflower seeds, soaked and toasted if possible (page 40)
½ teaspoon ground cinnamon
Sweetener is optional, 0 to 2 tablespoons sweetener
    (See options on page 18. Brown sweetener is tasty in this.)
¼ cup berries, such as raspberries, blueberries, strawberries, etc.

- In a pan on the stove, heat the milk to boiling.

- Grind the flaxseeds in a hand-held grinder or super-blender. Place them in a heat-proof cereal bowl.

- Add to the bowl coconut, nuts, cinnamon, and sweetener, if using.

- Pour the milk into the bowl and stir well. Sprinkle berries on top and enjoy.

Gluten-free	Dairy-free	Egg-free	Meat-free	Tree Nut-free	Vegan	Diabetic-friendly	Candida-friendly	High-protein	10 minutes or less
●	●	●	●		●	●	●		●

FLAX OATMEAL WITH BANANA

This super-easy Paleo porridge tastes like oatmeal with cinnamon, banana, and nuts. It's the quickest breakfast in town and will hold hunger at bay all morning. Flaxseeds are a powerful superfood, loaded with high omega-3 nutrition. Due to their delicate oils, flaxseeds must be consumed immediately after grinding, in order to avoid free radicals, and should never be cooked. Raw flaxseed meal is delicious—just stir the ingredients together, and in 10 minutes they'll expand to thicken the porridge. For a powerful nutrition boost, top it with High-Protein Coconut Milk (page 35) or High-Protein Nut Milk (page 37).

YIELD: Serves one • EQUIPMENT: Hand-held grinder or super-blender

2 tablespoons whole flaxseeds
½ cup unsweetened coconut milk (page 35) or nut milk (page 36)
1 tablespoon almond butter (page 38)
1 tablespoon hemp nuts
¼ teaspoon ground cinnamon
½ teaspoon vanilla
A pinch of ground nutmeg
A pinch of unprocessed salt
About 1 teaspoon sweetener to taste (see options on page 18)
½ ripe banana, sliced
⅓ cup nuts or seeds, walnuts pecans, almonds, Brazil nuts,
    pumpkin seeds, sunflower seeds, cashews, and/or hazelnuts,
    soaked and crisped or toasted if possible (page 40)

- Grind the flaxseeds in a hand-held grinder or super-blender.

- In a cereal bowl, stir together the ground flaxseeds, coconut milk, almond butter, hemp nuts, cinnamon, vanilla, nutmeg, salt, and sweetener. Slice the banana on top and sprinkle with nuts.

- Allow the cereal to rest for 10 minutes so the flaxseed can soften and thicken your cereal. Go get dressed, and your breakfast will be ready!

Gluten-free	Dairy-free	Egg-free	Meat-free	Tree Nut–free	Vegan	Diabetic-friendly	Candida-friendly	High-protein	10 minutes or less
●	●	●	●		●	●	●		●

COCONUT PANNA COTTA
WITH HONEY AND WALNUTS

This delicious custard is my go-to dairy-free yogurt substitute. It's a snap to make, way quicker than the original Italian recipe. It takes 5 minutes to prepare and 30 minutes to firm up. Or make it the night before, and your "yogurt" breakfast is ready when you wake up. Instead of gelatin, it uses agar powder, which will thicken the custard without being chilled (see Ingredients, page 9).

YIELD: 2 ramekins or mugs

¼ cup walnuts, soaked and toasted if possible (page 40)
1¾ cups thick full-fat unsweetened coconut milk (page 13)
½ teaspoon agar powder
2 teaspoons arrowroot flour
2 teaspoons raw honey, or 1 tablespoon zero-carb sweetener, optional (see options on page 18)

2 teaspoons lemon juice
1 teaspoon vanilla
Zest of 1 orange (optional)

GARNISH:
1 handful of walnuts
2 teaspoons raw honey or 1 tablespoon zero-carb sweetener (see page 18 for options)
A pinch of ground cinnamon

- Put the walnuts in the bottom of two ramekins or mugs.

- In a small saucepan away from heat, whisk together the coconut milk, agar powder, arrowroot, honey, lemon juice, vanilla, and orange zest, if using. Don't worry if the honey doesn't quite dissolve—it will melt soon. Bring to a slow boil over medium heat, stirring frequently. Remove from the heat immediately and pour into the ramekins over the walnuts. Chill 30 minutes. Top with walnuts, honey, and cinnamon in the morning.

VARIATION: Coconut Panna Cotta with Berries and Nuts
Add a handful of berries to the empty cups and sprinkle them on top.

Gluten-free	Dairy-free	Egg-free	Meat-free	Tree Nut–free	Vegan	Diabetic-friendly	Candida-friendly	High-protein	10 minutes or less
●	●	●	●		●	●	●		

CAULIFLOWER RICE PUDDING

If you love rice pudding and are feeling grain-deprived, this pudding is for you. When combined with coconut milk, the unlikely ingredient of cauliflower creates a pudding that is rich, creamy, and surprisingly similar to my mom's rice pudding.

YIELD: 1½ cups; serves one • **EQUIPMENT:** A food processor or a high-speed blender is helpful but not required

¾ cup full-fat unsweetened coconut milk (page 13)
2 tablespoons shredded unsweetened coconut
A splash of vanilla
A pinch of unprocessed salt
¼ teaspoon ground cinnamon
⅛ teaspoon ground or freshly grated nutmeg
1 cup (about 135 grams) fresh, raw cauliflower, riced (see Tip)
2 tablespoons coconut oil
1 to 3 teaspoons sweetener to taste (see options on page 18)

- In a small saucepan over low heat, place the coconut milk, coconut, vanilla, salt, cinnamon, and nutmeg. Bring to a boil stirring, and then turn the heat way down to a very low simmer. Cover and cook for 6 minutes on very low heat.

- "Rice" the cauliflower in a food processor or high-speed blender. Add riced cauliflower and coconut oil to the saucepan. Stir gently, bring to a boil again, cover and cook on very low heat for 2 to 6 more minutes. Cook until the shredded coconut is easy to chew, without overcooking the cauliflower, and the texture is like old-fashioned rice pudding.

- Sweeten to taste. Pour into a serving bowl. Serve warm or cold, garnished with cinnamon.

Tip: To rice cauliflower, put chunks of cauliflower into the bowl of your food processor or blender and pulse until the cauliflower is in small, rice-size pieces. Or you can grate it fine with a box grater.

Gluten-free	Dairy-free	Egg-free	Meat-free	Tree Nut–free	Vegan	Diabetic-friendly	Candida-friendly	High-protein	10 minutes or less
●	●	●	●	●	●	●	●		●

KASHA WITH BACON AND MUSHROOMS

This is a wonderfully warm, savory breakfast, with the irresistible flavor of bacon. Kasha means porridge in Russian, and peasants have lived on it for centuries. Buckwheat is neither a grain nor a grass, but rather a fruit seed related to rhubarb. This makes it an ideal Paleo food that's gluten- and grain-free. Like all seeds and nuts, it is best soaked overnight. Bacon adds a tantalizing flavor. Look for non-GMO, sugar-free bacon, if possible.

YIELD: Serves two

1½ cups dry, raw buckwheat groats, soaked overnight (see directions)
3 strips bacon, cooked and chopped, or 3 tablespoons
    Homemade Bacon Bits (page 42)
½ onion, chopped
1 cup fresh mushrooms (any type), sliced, or 1 ounce dried mushrooms,
    soaked in water to rehydrate
2 cups filtered water
Unprocessed salt and pepper to taste

- Place the buckwheat and 2 cups water in a glass bowl. Cover and soak for 8 hours or overnight at room temperature. In the morning, rinse well, drain, and set aside.

- In a large skillet over medium heat, cook the bacon for 1 minute. Add the onions and sauté until they begin to soften, about 3 minutes. Add the mushrooms and sauté for 2 minutes.

- Add the buckwheat and 2 cups filtered water. Season with salt and pepper, remembering the bacon is salty, too. Bring to a boil. Reduce the heat to very low and simmer for about 30 minutes, stirring occasionally until the buckwheat has cooked through. Add a bit more water if necessary to keep it from sticking.

- Pour into two cereal bowls and enjoy!

Gluten-free	Dairy-free	Egg-free	Meat-free	Tree Nut–free	Vegan	Diabetic-friendly	Candida-friendly	High-protein	10 minutes or less
●	●	●		●		●			

5

GRIDDLE GOODIES

"Nature itself is the best physician."
—Hippocrates, 460–400 BCE, Greek physician

I have a passion for pancakes! Gluten-free pancakes and waffles are everywhere these days. However grain-free griddle goodies are a completely new breed of healthy breakfast treat. There's no need for deprivation when you're eating Paleo. All you need is an open mind and a touch of imagination to reinvent your former decadent favorites into truly healthy breakfasts. Conventional pancakes are made with refined flours that are high in carbs, such as wheat, rice, potato, or tapioca, and sweeteners that will ultimately land on your waistline. However these recipes are extremely low-carb and guilt-free, with a fraction of the carbs and sugars in conventional recipes. That's because they're made with low-carb, grain-free almond meal, coconut meat, and zero-carb sweeteners.

These Paleo pancakes and waffles are made with 100 percent hunt-and-gather ingredients, yet they're hardly caveman food. Children and adults love Blueberry Pancakes (page 117) and gobble them down without guessing they're packed with nutrient-dense ingredients. Squash Bacon Waffles with Pecans (page 129) are a double indulgence with Hot Caramel Sauce (page 248). The recipes are designed to be easy for a beginning cook, so you can enjoy them in 15 minutes or less. Now you can have pancakes or waffles any day of the week, not just a special weekend treat.

Grain-free pancakes tend to be slightly denser than conventional ones, but they have even more flavor. Try whipping up a short stack and top your creations with luscious syrups in Chapter 11, such as Blackberry Sauce (page 243), Maple Flavor Syrup (page 246), or my favorite, Ginger Cardamom Syrup (page 247). I find that people enjoy Paleo pancakes just as much or even more than those sticky-sweet flapjacks we used to eat.

10 Tips for Perfect Paleo Pancakes and Waffles

1. Get ready. Have your toppings ready to go so you can enjoy hot pancakes or waffles without waiting. Set up a condiment selection on the table, and let everyone add their favorite toppings. Prepare a baking sheet or heatproof platter to keep cooked pancakes or waffles warm, covered with a cloth. Put it in the oven and preheat it to 200°F.

2. Take your time. There's no rush. Measure ingredients carefully. Here's one place to follow instructions.

3. Use a wadded paper towel to apply coconut oil evenly to your skillet, griddle, or waffle maker. Repeat for each batch of waffles or pancakes.

4. Temperature is the #1 key. You want the heat hot, but not too hot. If the heat is too hot or too cold, the pancakes or waffles may scorch, or they won't rise. Start with a medium-high heat. If your pancake griddle has a temperature control, heat it to 375°F. For waffles, follow the manufacturer's instructions.

5. For pancakes, 3 to 4 tablespoons batter is best. Use a ¼ cup almost full to pour the batter onto the hot griddle. Work quickly and leave space between each one. For waffles, a ⅓ cup measure is perfect.

Do a test run with a sacrificial pancake or waffle. See how it comes out and adjust the temperature up or down as needed. Your heat is too high if they're brown on the outside and still wet on the inside. Your heat is too low if they just sit there for 2 minutes with no change in color—they should be browning. And don't worry—if your first pancakes or waffles aren't perfect; you'll get better with practice.

6. Don't press your pancakes or waffles. Pressing will just make them heavy and flat, instead of light and fluffy.

7. When to flip a pancake: Let the pancake cook until the edges start to look dry. Don't move the pancake before this, as it may break. Grain-free pancakes don't always do the bubble thing. If you see bubbles form on the top, wait for most of them to break. Or peek at the underside—when it's golden brown and the pancake is firm enough to move, it's time to flip.

8. How to flip a pancake: Use a thin spatula and carefully slide it under the pancake. Flipping delicate grain-free pancakes often requires two spatulas, one in each hand to gently lift the pancake onto one of the spatulas. Then with a flick of your wrist, quickly flip the pancake. Let the pancake cook for another minute or two. The second side will not brown as completely as the first.

9. When one comes out right, repeat for the rest. When you're satisfied that you've reached the perfect temperature for your pancake skillet or waffle maker, go ahead and fill it to make more. In the case of pancakes, leave a little room between them for expansion and comfortable flipping.

10. Don't wait—eat them now. Pancakes and waffles are best eaten fresh and hot, so you can enjoy their crispy, fluffy goodness. This may mean that you're working at the stove while the rest of the family digs in.

BANANA NUT PANCAKES WITH CARDAMOM

I love the aroma of fresh banana cooking with cardamom! Green bananas are a great find for low-carb fans, to start your morning out with balanced blood sugar. They're in stark contrast to the high sugars and carbs in ripe bananas. The banana flavor combines deliciously with Ginger Cardamom Syrup (page 247) or Maple Flavor Syrup (page 246). Freeze leftovers on a paper plate in a freezer bag with a piece of parchment paper between each pancake for up to 3 months and reheat for a quick meal.

YIELD: Nine pancakes; serves two • **EQUIPMENT:** A food processor is helpful but not required

1 green banana, mashed (about ½ cup)
½ tablespoon lemon juice
¼ cup almond butter (page 38)
2 large eggs
1 to 2 tablespoons unsweetened
   coconut milk (page 35)
½ teaspoon vanilla
½ cup almond meal
2 tablespoons arrowroot flour
1½ tablespoons coconut flour

¼ teaspoon baking soda
⅛ teaspoon unprocessed salt
¼ teaspoon ground cardamom
⅛ teaspoon ground cinnamon
2 tablespoons raw honey or
   3 tablespoons zero-carb sweetener
   (see page 18 for options)
¼ cup chopped nuts, soaked and toasted
   if possible (page 40)
Coconut oil for frying

- Prepare the syrup or any toppings desired.

- In a food processor or mixing bowl, place the banana, lemon juice, almond butter, eggs, coconut milk, and vanilla. Mix well.

- To the mixture in the processor, add almond meal, arrowroot, coconut flour, baking soda, salt, cardamom, cinnamon, and honey and mix briefly.

- Pulse in the nuts so they remain in large pieces.

- See "10 Tips for Perfect Paleo Pancakes and Waffles" (page 114). Use a wadded paper towel to lightly grease a large nonstick skillet or griddle with coconut oil. Heat on medium-high heat until a drop of water sizzles when flicked onto the pan. Then you know it is ready.

continues

continued

- For each pancake, use a scant ¼ cup measure to pour 3 tablespoons of batter onto the skillet. You should be able to fit two to three pancakes in a large skillet.

- Cook on the first side for 2 to 3 minutes. Flip and cook on the other side until browned, for 1 to 2 minutes more. If they're delicate, use two spatulas to flip. Place finished pancakes on a serving plate covered with a towel. Repeat until all the batter is cooked. Serve with fruit and your favorite syrup or toppings.

Gluten-free	Dairy-free	Egg-free	Meat-free	Tree Nut–free	Vegan	Diabetic-friendly	Candida-friendly	High-protein	10 minutes or less
●	●		●			●	●		

BLUEBERRY PANCAKES

I can't live without blueberry pancakes. These are grain-free, tree nut–free, quick, and scrumptious. Blueberry pancakes taste even better with easy Berrylicious Sauce (page 243), and you can make the whole breakfast in 15 minutes or less. Luscious and low-carb, coconut butter gives them a rich, subtle sweetness. Leftover pancakes freeze well in a resealable bag with parchment paper between the layers. Pull them out when needed and heat briefly in a pan for an easy breakfast.

YIELD: Twelve pancakes; serves four • **EQUIPMENT:** A food processor is helpful but not required

½ cup almond meal
½ teaspoon baking soda
¼ teaspoon unprocessed salt
½ cup (113 grams) Coconut Butter (page 33); if mixing by hand, soften butter by placing the container in a bowl of warm water
4 large eggs, at room temperature

2 teaspoons vanilla
1 teaspoon apple cider vinegar
¼ cup unsweetened coconut milk (page 35), or a bit more if needed
About ½ cup sweetener to taste (see options on page 18)
1 cup fresh blueberries (or ¾ cup frozen hard)

• Prepare Berrylicious Sauce and your favorite pancake toppings. Get out a large nonstick skillet or griddle.

• In a food processor or mixing bowl, place the almond meal, baking soda, and salt. Mix well. Add coconut butter and mix to a thick paste.

• Add to the mixture: eggs, vanilla, vinegar, and coconut milk. Process briefly. Slightly lumpy batter is no problem. Add sweetener to taste, and mix again. Add frozen blueberries to the batter and stir them in with a rubber spatula so they stay whole. The batter should be thick and pourable. To thin it, stir in a bit more coconut milk until it is barely pourable. To thicken it, add almond meal one tablespoon at a time. See "10 Tips for Perfect Paleo Pancakes and Waffles" (page 114). Use a wadded paper towel to lightly grease a large nonstick skillet or griddle with coconut oil. Heat on medium-high heat until a drop of water sizzles when flicked onto the pan. Then you know it is ready.

continues

- For each pancake, use a scant ¼ cup measure to pour 3 tablespoons of batter onto the skillet. You should be able to fit two to three pancakes in a large skillet.

- Cook on the first side for 2 to 3 minutes. Flip and cook on the other side until browned, for 1 to 2 minutes more. If they're delicate, use two spatulas to flip. Place finished pancakes on a serving plate covered with a towel. Repeat until all the batter is cooked. Serve with fruit and your favorite syrup or toppings.

Gluten-free	Dairy-free	Egg-free	Meat-free	Tree Nut–free	Vegan	Diabetic-friendly	Candida-friendly	High-protein	10 minutes or less
●	●		●			●	●		

TRADITIONAL PLANTAIN PANCAKES

A traditional favorite breakfast in Central and South America, these rich plantain griddle cakes taste amazing with Orange Maple Syrup (page 246) or Orange Honey Butter (page 251). Look for a green plantain if you can, for a lower carb count. These are easiest to make in a food processor. However you can also make them by hand, mixing dry and wet ingredients separately—mash the plantain and stir everything together. Freeze leftovers in a resealable plastic bag with parchment paper between the pancakes. Then pull them out and reheat in a pan for an instant breakfast.

YIELD: Ten to twelve pancakes; serves four • **EQUIPMENT:** A food processor is helpful but not required

½ cup almond meal
2 tablespoons coconut flour
½ teaspoon baking soda
⅛ teaspoon unprocessed salt
½ teaspoon ground cinnamon
1 plantain, preferably green
2 tablespoons almond butter
2 large eggs (110 grams)
¼ cup coconut milk (page 35) or almond milk (page 36)
Sweetener is optional, 0 to 3 tablespoons (see options on page 18)
2 tablespoons coconut oil for frying

- Prepare your favorite syrup.

- In a food processor with the "S" blade place the almond meal, coconut flour, baking soda, salt, cinnamon, plantain, almond butter, eggs, and milk. Sweeten to taste—this will depend on the flavor of your plantain.

- Process well until the plantain is liquefied. Texture and flavor will vary depending on your plantain. If the batter is too runny, add a bit more almond meal. If it is too thick, add more milk a teaspoon at a time until it is a thick, pourable batter. If you add too much liquid, the pancakes will fall apart.

- See "10 Tips for Perfect Paleo Pancakes and Waffles" (page 114). Use a wadded paper towel to lightly grease a large nonstick skillet or griddle with coconut oil. Heat on medium heat until a drop of water sizzles when flicked onto the pan. Then you know it is ready.

continues

- For each pancake, use a scant ¼ cup measure to pour 3 tablespoons of batter onto the skillet. You should be able to fit two to three pancakes in a large skillet.

- Cook for 2 to 4 minutes until the underside is lightly browned, and the pancake is firm enough to flip. Flip and cook on the other side until browned, for 2 to 3 minutes more. I suggest using two spatulas to flip, so they don't break. Place finished pancakes on a serving plate covered with a towel. Repeat until all the batter is cooked. Serve with fruit and your favorite syrup or toppings.

Gluten-free	Dairy-free	Egg-free	Meat-free	Tree Nut–free	Vegan	Diabetic-friendly	Candida-friendly	High-protein	10 minutes or less
●	●		●			●	●		

ZUCCHINI PANCAKES

With onion, garlic, and a hint of Parmesan cheese, these *Frittelle di Zucchini* are a little taste of Italy! These are especially delicious with Paleo Sour Cream (page 256). You can freeze leftovers in a resealable bag with parchment paper between the pancakes. Then pull them out and reheat for a hot breakfast in minutes.

YIELD: Nine pancakes • **EQUIPMENT NEEDED:** None

1 medium zucchini, coarsely grated (about ¾ pound), including the peel
½ teaspoon unprocessed salt
2 large eggs
2 green onions, chopped
Black pepper to taste
2 tablespoons (28 grams) Coconut Butter (page 33),
    softened (place the container in a bowl of warm water), or any nut butter
1 tablespoon lemon juice
1 tablespoon nutritional yeast
1 tablespoon chopped fresh herbs, such as basil, parsley, or tarragon
1 clove garlic, chopped or crushed (optional)
3 tablespoons almond meal, and 2 more if necessary
2 tablespoons onion flakes (optional)
2 tablespoons coconut oil for frying

- Coarsely grate the zucchini into a large mixing bowl using the large grating side of a box grater. I find grating by hand is quick for this, or you can use a food processor.

- It's helpful to draw moisture out of the zucchini so the pancakes will hold together. Stir ¼ teaspoon of the salt into the zucchini and put it in a large strainer over a bowl. Press the zucchini with a spatula to release water. Allow it to sit for a few minutes while the excess water drains out.

- In a medium mixing bowl, beat the eggs. Whisk in the green onions, remaining salt, pepper, coconut butter, lemon juice, nutritional yeast, herbs, garlic, almond meal, and onion flakes, if using.

- Press the zucchini again to squeeze out any excess water. Add it to the egg mixture and stir well. If the batter is too thin for pancakes, add 2 more tablespoons almond meal.

continues

continued

- See "10 Tips for Perfect Paleo Pancakes and Waffles" (page 114). Use a wadded paper towel to lightly grease a large nonstick skillet or griddle with coconut oil. Heat on medium-high heat until a drop of water sizzles when flicked onto the pan. Then you know it is ready.

- For each pancake, use a scant ¼ cup measure to pour 3 tablespoons of batter onto the skillet. You should be able to fit two to three pancakes in a large skillet.

- Cook until the underside is golden brown, for 2 to 3 minutes. Flip and cook on the other side until browned, for 1 to 2 minutes more. If they're delicate, use two spatulas to flip. Place finished pancakes on a serving plate covered with a towel. Repeat until all the batter is cooked. Serve with fruit and your favorite syrup or toppings.

Gluten-free	Dairy-free	Egg-free	Meat-free	Tree Nut-free	Vegan	Diabetic-friendly	Candida-friendly	High-protein	10 minutes or less
●	●		●			●	●		

SWEET POTATO LATKES

The very best latkes that I have ever tasted are made with sweet potatoes. We know potato pancakes as a traditional Hanukkah dish, and they're also a classic favorite throughout Eastern Europe. Serve them with mellow Paleo Sour Cream (page 256). It's quickest to fry them on the stove top, or you can bake them for equally delicious results. Freeze leftovers in a resealable bag with parchment paper between the pancakes. Defrost and reheat them for a lovely breakfast in minutes.

YIELD: Twenty pancakes; serves four • **EQUIPMENT:** A food processor with grater is helpful but not required

1 recipe Paleo Sour Cream (page 256)
1 medium sweet potato, peeled
1 Granny Smith apple, peeled and cored
1 small to medium onion
1 cup shredded unsweetened coconut

½ cup arrowroot flour
3 large eggs
1 teaspoon unprocessed salt
Black pepper to taste
3 green onions, finely chopped
Coconut oil for frying

- Prepare the Paleo Sour Cream.

- Coarsely grate the sweet potato, apple, and onion in a food processor or with a hand grater.

- In a mixing bowl, mix the shredded coconut, arrowroot, eggs, salt, pepper, and green onions.

- Add the grated potato mixture and stir until well combined.

- Use a wadded paper towel to lightly grease a large nonstick skillet or griddle with coconut oil. Heat on medium heat until a drop of water sizzles when flicked onto the pan. Then you know it is ready.

- See "10 Tips for Perfect Paleo Pancakes and Waffles" (page 114). For each pancake, use a scant ¼ cup measure to put three tablespoons of batter onto the skillet. You should be able to fit two to three pancakes in a large skillet. I use two pans for faster cooking. Press them down with a spatula into about 4-inch rounds. Fry each one for 4 to 5 minutes on each side, or until they are barely a golden brown color. Place finished latkes on a serving dish covered with a towel to keep warm. These are equally satisfying baked on a parchment-covered baking sheet for 25 to 35 minutes at 350°F.

Gluten-free	Dairy-free	Egg-free	Meat-free	Tree Nut-free	Vegan	Diabetic-friendly	Candida-friendly	High-protein	10 minutes or less
●	●		●	●		●	●		

SWEET POTATO PANCAKES

A traditional Southern food, sweet potatoes are high in vitamin B_6 and beta-carotene. They contain almost twice as much fiber as white potatoes, which gives them a "slow burning" quality and helps set up level energy patterns all day. Almond meal and almond butter add a pleasant mellow flavor and make these pancakes high-protein and low-carb. My favorite topping for them is Orange Honey Butter (page 251).

YIELD: Twelve 4-inch pancakes; serves four • **EQUIPMENT:** A food processor is helpful. If you don't have one, use cooked, mashed sweet potato and mix the batter by hand.

1 recipe Orange Honey Butter
   (page 251)
2 cups sweet potato, peeled and cubed
¾ cup almond meal
⅓ cup almond butter (page 38)
3 large eggs
¼ teaspoon unprocessed salt

1 teaspoon vanilla
1 teaspoon ground cinnamon
About 2 tablespoons sweetener to taste
   (See options on page 18. I especially
   like half brown sweetener in this.)
1 tablespoon coconut oil for frying

- Prepare Orange Honey Butter, if desired.

- In a food processor or mixing bowl, place all the ingredients: sweet potato, almond meal, almond butter, eggs, salt, vanilla, cinnamon, and sweetener. Process well, about one minute, or until the sweet potato is liquefied.

- See "10 Tips for Perfect Paleo Pancakes and Waffles" (page 114). Use a wadded paper towel to lightly grease a large nonstick skillet or griddle with coconut oil. Heat on medium-high heat until a drop of water sizzles when flicked onto the pan. Then you know it is ready.

- For each pancake, use a scant ¼ cup measure to pour 3 tablespoons of batter onto the skillet. You should be able to fit two to three pancakes in a large skillet.

- Cook until the top of the pancake has a few bubbles and some of them have burst—2 to 3 minutes. Flip and cook on the other side until browned, for 1 to 2 minutes more. If they're delicate, use two spatulas to flip. Place finished pancakes on a serving plate covered with a towel. Repeat until all the batter is cooked. Serve with fruit and your favorite syrup or toppings.

Gluten-free	Dairy-free	Egg-free	Meat-free	Tree Nut-free	Vegan	Diabetic-friendly	Candida-friendly	High-protein	10 minutes or less
●	●		●			●	●		

CHOCOLATE BROWNIE
SUPERFOOD WAFFLES

Looks like a waffle, tastes like a waffle. But, ah, how appearances can deceive. What tastes like a decadently rich sweet is secretly a high-protein superfood breakfast. These are quick to make and super-luscious with Blackberry Sauce (page 243). Freeze leftovers wrapped individually in a freezer bag. Then pop the frozen waffles in the toaster when you need a quick breakfast.

YIELD: Seven to eight waffles; serves four • **EQUIPMENT:** A food processor is helpful but not required; waffle iron

½ cup (113 grams) Coconut Butter (page 33); if mixing by hand, soften butter by placing the container in a bowl of warm water

⅓ cup pure cacao powder, or ½ cup carob powder

¼ teaspoon unprocessed salt

¼ teaspoon baking soda

½ apple, cored, in chunks with the peel (if mixing by hand, grate the apple)

⅓ cup almond butter (page 38)

2 tablespoons coconut oil

3 large eggs (165 grams)

2 teaspoons vanilla

Zest of 1 orange (optional)

About ⅔ cup sweetener to taste (see options on page 18)

Optional superfood additions (see list)

½ cup liquid or more as needed to thin batter, such as coconut milk (page 35), almond milk (page 36), or filtered water

OPTIONAL SUPERFOOD ADDITIONS:

3 tablespoons chopped nuts (almonds, pecans, etc.), soaked and toasted if possible (page 40)

2 tablespoons of your favorite protein powder

1 teaspoon nutritional yeast

1 teaspoon chlorella powder or green powder

1 tablespoon soaked hiziki or wakame seaweed

1 tablespoon maca powder

1 dropper-full ChlorOxygen

¼ teaspoon bee pollen

continues

- Prepare your toppings. Heat a waffle iron.

- In a food processor or mixing bowl, place the coconut butter, cacao powder, salt, and baking soda. Process until there are no lumps.

- To the ingredients in the processor, add the apple, almond butter, coconut oil, eggs, vanilla, zest, if using, and sweetener. Process well until the apple is completely liquefied.

- Add your favorite superfoods, all optional. Process well. The batter will be quite thick. Add a small amount of liquid slowly until it is a thick batter that you can just barely pour. If you have to spoon it in, it is too thick, and the waffles will be a bit heavy.

- Dip a basting brush in a jar of coconut oil and lightly brush the warm waffle iron. Spread ¼ cup batter over each iron. Close the lid, and cook per the manufacturer's instructions, usually for 3 to 5 minutes, until the waffle iron indicator shows that cooking is complete, or no more steam comes out. Open the lid and check the waffles. If they aren't fully cooked close the lid and wait a minute.

- Waffles are done when they're crispy and you can pull them out with a fork or a pair of tongs. Take care not to scratch the nonstick surface. Serve immediately or transfer the finished waffles to a platter covered with a cloth in the oven set at 200°F to keep warm.

- Enjoy the waffles hot with your favorite toppings.

Gluten-free	Dairy-free	Egg-free	Meat-free	Tree Nut-free	Vegan	Diabetic-friendly	Candida-friendly	High-protein	10 minutes or less
●	●		●			●	●		

PECAN WAFFLES

These crisp and delicate waffles will melt in your mouth. I like them with Maple Flavor Syrup (page 246) or Maple Pecan Syrup (page 246). Crunchy and flavorful, pecans are also a rich source of vitamin E and antioxidants that benefit the heart, lower bad cholesterol levels, and protect against inflammation. Freeze leftover waffles in a resealable bag with parchment paper between each waffle. Pull them out whenever you need them, and pop them in a toaster to defrost.

YIELD: Seven to eight waffles; serves four • **EQUIPMENT:** Food processor and waffle iron

⅔ cup almond meal

½ teaspoon baking soda

1 tablespoon nutritional yeast

¼ teaspoon unprocessed salt

⅔ cup (151 grams) Coconut Butter (page 33); if mixing by hand, soften butter by placing the container in a bowl of warm water

4 large eggs at room temperature

2 teaspoons vanilla

2 tablespoons lemon juice

½ teaspoon apple cider vinegar

About ⅓ cup sweetener to taste (see options on page 18)

¾ cup chopped pecans, soaked and toasted if possible (page 40)

- Prepare your choice of toppings. Heat a waffle iron.

- In a dry food processor or mixing bowl, place the almond meal, baking soda, nutritional yeast, and salt. Mix well. Add the coconut butter and mix to a thick paste.

- To the mixture in the bowl, add the eggs, vanilla, lemon juice, and vinegar. Process well. Add the sweetener to taste and mix again. Don't worry if your batter is slightly lumpy—it will still turn out just fine. Pulse in the pecans.

- Dip a basting brush in a jar of coconut oil and lightly brush the warm waffle iron. Spread ¼ cup batter over each iron. Close the lid, and cook per the manufacturer's instructions, usually for 3 to 5 minutes, until the waffle iron indicator shows that cooking is complete, or no more steam comes out of the waffle iron. Open the lid and check the waffles. If they aren't fully cooked close the lid and wait a minute.

- Waffles are done when they're crispy, barely golden brown, and you can pull them out with a fork or pair of tongs. Take care not to scratch the nonstick surface. Serve immediately or transfer the finished waffles to a platter covered with a cloth in the oven set at 200°F to keep warm.

- Enjoy the waffles hot with your favorite toppings.

Gluten-free	Dairy-free	Egg-free	Meat-free	Tree Nut-free	Vegan	Diabetic-friendly	Candida-friendly	High-protein	10 minutes or less
●	●		●			●	●	●	

SOUR CREAM WAFFLES

These waffles are delicate, crispy, and full of sour cream flavor. They're dairy-free; the rich taste comes from coconut butter and lemon. They're also tree nut–free for those people with food allergies. I love these with Orange Honey Butter (page 251) or Maple Pecan Syrup (page 246). You can freeze leftovers in a resealable bag with parchment paper between each waffle then heat them in the toaster for a quick hot breakfast.

YIELD: Eight waffles; serves four • **EQUIPMENT:** A food processor is helpful but not required; a waffle iron

⅔ cup arrowroot flour
½ teaspoon baking soda
¼ teaspoon unprocessed salt
1 tablespoon nutritional yeast (optional)
⅔ cup (151 grams) Coconut Butter (page 33); if mixing by hand, soften butter by placing the container in a bowl of warm water

4 large eggs at room temperature
2 teaspoons pure vanilla
2 tablespoons lemon juice
About ½ cup sweetener to taste (see options on page 18)

- Prepare your choice of toppings. Heat a waffle iron.
- In a dry food processor or mixing bowl, place the arrowroot, baking soda, salt, and nutritional yeast, if using. Mix until smooth. Add the coconut butter and mix to a thick paste.
- To the ingredients in the food processor, add the eggs, vanilla, lemon juice, and sweetener to taste. Mix briefly. If you're working by hand, beat in these ingredients and stir well.
- Don't worry if your batter is slightly lumpy—it will turn out fine.
- Dip a basting brush in a jar of coconut oil and lightly brush the warm waffle iron. Spread ¼ cup batter over each iron. Close the lid, and cook per the manufacturer's instructions, usually for 3 to 5 minutes, until the waffle iron indicator shows that cooking is complete, or no more steam comes out of the waffle iron. Open the lid and check the waffles. If they aren't fully cooked, close the lid and wait a minute.
- Waffles are done when they're crispy, barely golden brown, and you can pull them out with a fork or pair of tongs. Take care not to scratch the nonstick surface. Serve immediately or transfer the finished waffles to a platter covered with a cloth in the oven set at 200°F to keep warm.
- Enjoy the waffles hot with your favorite toppings.

Gluten-free	Dairy-free	Egg-free	Meat-free	Tree Nut–free	Vegan	Diabetic-friendly	Candida-friendly	High-protein	10 minutes or less
●	●		●	●		●	●		

SQUASH BACON WAFFLES WITH PECANS

While this combo may seem very autumnal, squash and bacon make a tantalizing combination any time of year. These pancakes are so easy, especially with precubed squash from the grocery store—it can be raw or cooked. Serve with Hot Caramel Sauce (page 248) or Orange Honey Butter (page 251). Freeze leftover waffles in a resealable bag with parchment paper between the layers. Then pop them in the toaster for a quick hot breakfast.

YIELD: Eight waffles; serves four • **EQUIPMENT:** A food processor is helpful but not required; waffle iron

2 cups butternut squash, peeled and cubed
  (if mixing by hand, cooked and mashed)
1 cup almond meal
2 tablespoons arrowroot flour
¼ teaspoon baking powder
⅓ cup coconut oil, melted
3 large eggs
¼ teaspoon unprocessed salt
1 teaspoon vanilla
1 teaspoon ground cinnamon
About ¼ cup sweetener to taste (see options on page 18)
⅓ cup chopped pecans (optional)
½ cup Homemade Bacon Bits (page 42), or 8 ounces natural sugar-free bacon,
  cooked and cut into ¼-inch squares (optional)
Your favorite applesauce or Hot Caramel Sauce (page 248)

- Preheat a waffle iron.

- In a food processor or mixing bowl, place the squash, almond meal, arrowroot, baking powder, coconut oil, eggs, salt, vanilla, cinnamon, and sweetener. Process well until the squash is liquefied and there are no bulky lumps. Add the pecans and pulse briefly so they remain in large pieces.

- Dip a basting brush in a jar of coconut oil and lightly brush the warm waffle iron. Spread ¼ cup batter over each iron. Sprinkle 1 tablespoon of bacon on top of each one. Close the lid, and cook per the manufacturer's instructions, usually for 3 to 5 minutes, until the waffle iron indicator shows that cooking is complete, or no more steam

continues

continued

comes out of the waffle iron. Open the lid and check the waffles. If they aren't fully cooked, close the lid and wait a minute.

- Waffles are done when they're crispy, barely golden brown, and you can pull them out with a fork or pair of tongs. Take care not to scratch the nonstick surface. Serve immediately or transfer the finished waffles to a platter covered with a cloth in the oven set at 200°F to keep warm.

- Enjoy the waffles hot with your favorite toppings.

Gluten-free	Dairy-free	Egg-free	Meat-free	Tree Nut–free	Vegan	Diabetic-friendly	Candida-friendly	High-protein	10 minutes or less
●	●					●	●	●	

CINNAMON SWIRL FRENCH TOAST

What makes this French toast so amazing? It's the bread you choose. My favorite is sumptuous Cinnamon Swirl Bread (page 56) or Fluffy White Sandwich Bread (page 55), a bit dried out. See photo insert. If your bread is already made, then French toast is the easiest breakfast around. Slice the bread thick so the pieces don't fall apart. Serve with your favorite syrup such as Ginger Cardamom Syrup (page 247) or Maple Flavor Syrup (page 246). Top with Paleo Butter (page 45) and Coconut Cream Topping (page 249), if desired. Yes, you can freeze leftover French toast with parchment paper between the slices and reheat for a quick breakfast.

YIELD: Serves two

2 large eggs, pasture organic
⅓ cup unsweetened full-fat coconut milk (page 13)
   or almond milk (page 36)
A pinch of ground cinnamon
1 teaspoon vanilla
4 thick slices of bread
1 tablespoon coconut oil for frying
½ cup berries (optional)

- Prepare the toppings. Get out a baking sheet or heatproof platter to keep finished French toast warm, covered with a cloth. Put it an oven preheated to 200°F.

- In a small mixing bowl, whisk together the eggs, milk, cinnamon, and vanilla. Pour it into a shallow, wide dish. Dip the bread slices into the dish. Let each one soak briefly, flip them over with a spatula and let them soak again. Don't let the bread soak so much that it falls apart.

- Use a wadded paper towel to lightly grease a large nonstick skillet or griddle with coconut oil. Heat on medium-high heat until a drop of water sizzles when flicked onto the pan. Then you know it is ready.

- Using a spatula, carefully put the soaked bread into the skillet. Fry briefly on each side until golden brown, about 2 minutes per side. Repeat for each slice.

- Serve immediately or transfer the finished pieces to a platter covered with a cloth in the oven set at 200°F to keep warm. Serve immediately with your favorite butter spread, syrup, and berries, if using.

continues

continued

VARIATION: Baked French Toast

This version can be prepped the night before and baked in the morning. It saves time on a busy schedule and tastes equally wonderful.

In a medium mixing bowl, whisk together the eggs, milk, cinnamon, and vanilla.

Pour the egg mixture into a greased 9 x 5-inch baking pan. Place the bread slices into the egg mixture so they're completely covered. Refrigerate for one hour or overnight.

The next morning, preheat the oven to 375°F. Bake the slices for 30 minutes, or until firm and golden on the top. Serve with your favorite toppings.

Gluten-free	Dairy-free	Egg-free	Meat-free	Tree Nut–free	Vegan	Diabetic-friendly	Candida-friendly	High-protein	10 minutes or less
●	●		●	●		●	●		

PERFECT PALEO CREPES

I was amazed these crepes are so easy—just blend four ingredients and presto!—perfect crepes like Julia's! You can fill them, roll them, or fold them in a thousand ways. Try filling them with Turkey Sausage with Apple and Sage (page 238), Scrambled Eggs with Cheese (page 213), or sautéed mushrooms and Hollandaise Sauce (page 254). Make sweet crepes with Berrylicious Sauce (page 243). Or fill with sliced bananas, nuts, cacao nibs, and Coconut Cream Topping (page 249). Fill them with dinner leftovers. Make authentic Crepes Suzette by dipping your crepes in luscious Suzette Sauce (see variation below). Freeze crepes on a paper plate, stacked with parchment paper between them. Then pull them out and heat briefly in a pan for a quick breakfast.

YIELD: Eleven crepes • **EQUIPMENT:** Any blender or hand mixer is helpful but not required. An 8-inch skillet, nonstick if possible.

4 large eggs
4 tablespoons thin unsweetened coconut milk (page 35) or filtered water. If your coconut milk is thick, you can use half coconut milk and half filtered water.
2 tablespoons arrowroot flour
1 tablespoon olive oil
Sweetener is optional, 0 to 1 tablespoon (see options on page 18)
Coconut oil for frying

- Add all the ingredients to any blender. Blend well. If you don't have a blender, beat with a hand mixer or whisk very well by hand.

- Preheat an 8-inch pan over medium heat. Brush the pan with a bit of coconut oil before making each crepe.

- Use 3 tablespoons batter for each crepe, in a ¼-cup measure filled three-quarters full. The batter should be quite thin. If necessary, you can thin the batter with a little water. The first crepe is a test for the batter and the heat level, so don't be alarmed if it looks a little strange—it just takes time to fine-tune these variables. Adjust the heat if necessary.

- Pour the batter into the pan and twirl it around gently to coat the surface. Watch carefully, and the crepe will start to dry out on the sides, slightly pulling away from the pan, about 1 to 2 minutes. When the entire crepe can slide and pull away from the pan, release the edges with a spatula and flip it gently by grabbing the edges with your fingers. When the second side is gently browned, after about 1 minute, slip it onto a serving plate.

- Make all the crepes, putting them in a stack, and cover with a dry towel.

continues

VARIATION: Crepes Suzette
1 recipe Perfect Paleo Crepes (page 133)

ORANGE SAUCE:
1 orange
1 teaspoon lemon juice
3 to 5 tablespoons sweetener to taste (see options on page 18)
⅓ cup coconut oil, melted (put the jar in a bowl of warm water)
½ teaspoon nutritional yeast (optional, for buttery flavor)
Strawberries, sliced (optional garnish)
Oranges, peeled, sliced (optional garnish)

Prepare the crepes.

To make the sauce: Zest the entire orange into the blender. Cut away the white pith left on the orange with a sharp knife. Slice the orange, seeding as you go, and put the slices in the blender. Add the lemon juice, sweetener, coconut oil, and nutritional yeast, if using. Blend until liquefied. Then heat the sauce in an 8-inch skillet over low heat.

To assemble Crepes Suzette: Place each crepe one at a time in the warm sauce for a few seconds to soak up the sauce. Fold into quarters and place on plates. Garnish with strawberries and orange slices, if desired.

Gluten-free	Dairy-free	Egg-free	Meat-free	Tree Nut–free	Vegan	Diabetic-friendly	Candida-friendly	High-protein	10 minutes or less
●	●		●	●		●	●	●	●

APPLE FRITTERS

Quick and easy fritters are a delightful treat to wake up to. Granny Smith apples are low in fructose sugars, plus they're particularly high in antioxidants Vitamin C and flavonoids to help neutralize harmful free radicals. Apple fritters taste heavenly with Maple Flavor Syrup (page 246) or Ginger Cardamom Syrup (page 247). Freeze leftovers for up to 6 weeks with a piece of parchment paper between each fritter and reheat for a quick meal.

YIELD: Eight to nine fritters, 3 to 4 inches each; serves two • **EQUIPMENT:** A food processor or small blender is helpful but not required

2 large eggs
1 Granny Smith apple, unpeeled, cored, coarsely chopped (if mixing by hand, grated)
½ teaspoon vanilla
½ cup almond meal
⅛ teaspoon unprocessed salt
½ teaspoon ground cinnamon

¼ teaspoon baking soda
Brown sweetener is optional, 0 to 1½ tablespoons (see options on page 18)
¼ cup chopped nuts, such as almonds, walnuts, pecans, soaked and toasted if possible (page 40)
1 tablespoon coconut oil for frying

- Prepare syrup or any toppings desired.

- In a food processor, small blender, or mixing bowl, place the eggs, apple, and vanilla. Process until the apple and peels are as liquefied as possible.

- To the egg mixture, add the almond meal, salt, cinnamon, and baking soda. Choose your sweetener and sweetness level. Add and mix briefly. The batter should be fairly thick.

- Add the nuts and mix briefly so they remain in large pieces.

- In a large nonstick skillet, melt the coconut oil over medium heat. Flick a drop of water into the hot pan—when it sizzles, it's ready. Spoon the batter in small pancakes about 3 inches in diameter and allow it to spread. Cook on the first side, for 1 to 2 minutes, until the bottom is golden brown. Flip, and cook on the other side, about 1 minute. Adjust the heat if necessary. It's easiest to use two spatulas to flip them, as they're soft. Serve!

Gluten-free	Dairy-free	Egg-free	Meat-free	Tree Nut-free	Vegan	Diabetic-friendly	Candida-friendly	High-protein	10 minutes or less
●	●		●			●	●		

6

SWEET QUICK BREADS AND MUFFINS

"You don't have to cook fancy or complicated masterpieces—just good food from fresh ingredients."
—Julia Child

I enjoy reinventing traditional muffins and quick breads with low-carb, low-sugar foods, because it requires creative thinking to find new techniques and ingredients. When you taste the results, I hope you'll agree it's worth the effort.

One way this creative thinking has manifested is the use of coconut butter in these breads as a flour. Coconut butter is a whole, unprocessed food with a smooth, nongrainy texture and rich flavor. It has one-fourth the carbs of wheat flour or coconut flour. You can buy coconut butter in any healthy grocery. Or save a bundle making it yourself with a super-blender or food processor. See the recipe on page 33. Cold, solid coconut butter is easy to measure by weight, but

more difficult to accurately measure by the cup—the hard chunks just don't go into cups very well. However, softened coconut butter is more liquid, so it can be accurately measured in cups.

These coconut butter recipes are designed so you can mix by hand or use a food processor. Both methods work. If you're using a food processor, to save time you can weigh the hard coconut butter, add it to the food processor in chunks, and let the machine grind it for you. If you're mixing by hand or don't have a scale, you can first soften the coconut butter by placing the container in a bowl of very warm water for a few minutes. Then spoon the soft butter into a measuring cup and add it to your mix. You'll find a more inventive use of ingredients with the egg-free, grain-free muffins; these rely on a combination of chia seeds, apple pulp, and a surprise ingredient—agar powder. While they don't rise quite as much as standard refined flours with egg, they do rise a good amount—and taste delicious.

Grain-free baking is different than baking with traditional grains, and in some ways easier. For example, there's never any worry about overmixing the batter. Go ahead and mix it as much as you want—there's no gluten! To grease and flour muffin tins, first spread coconut oil into the cups with your fingers. Then use a fine-gauge strainer, tapping it lightly with a spoon, to sprinkle coconut flour evenly into the cups. When baking with coconut butter, remember that it is highly sensitive to temperature changes. It helps to start with your ingredients at room temperature. This is especially important for eggs—just immerse them for a few minutes in a bowl of warm water before adding them to the batter.

Here's a little-known secret to make grain-free muffins and quick breads rise faster: For a gorgeous muffin-top dome on muffins and quick breads, consider using this temperature trick: Preheat the oven to 400°F. Place the muffins or quick bread in the oven and immediately turn the heat down to 375°F. In 5 minutes turn it down to 350°F, and 5 minutes later, to 325°F for the remaining baking time. Grain-free muffins still don't rise as much as conventional muffins, but this really helps. It works so well, I wish they'd make ovens that do this automatically.

Finally, no matter which recipe you're making, the storage tips are pretty general for every recipe. These recipes make several loaves or muffins, just so you'll have leftovers. To store quick breads, slice the bread and cut small pieces of parchment paper to put between each slice. Then store in a freezer bag for breakfasts next week. To store muffins, wrap individually and put in a BPA-free storage container for a great grab-and-go breakfast.

BANANA BREAD

Here's a moist and tasty banana bread with a healthy surprise. Instead of yellow bananas, it uses green bananas. Don't worry, the bread isn't green, it just uses the unripe fruit, which has surprising health benefits. Green bananas contain resistant starch, which is not digested like other carbs. Instead it passes through the body unchanged like insoluble fiber—a great boon for weight control. Resistant starch also increases fat-burning, gives a sense of satiety, and reduces cravings. Green bananas are lower in fructose sugars than ripe ones, making them an all-around great start for the day. This bread tastes great with Paleo Cream Cheese (page 43).

YIELD: Three 4.5 x 2.5-inch mini loaves; two 7 x 3-inch loaves; one 9 x 5-inch loaf; or a 9-inch square pan • **EQUIPMENT:** A food processor is helpful but not required

1 cup almond meal
1 teaspoon baking soda
¼ heaping teaspoon unprocessed salt
1 tablespoon ground cinnamon
¼ teaspoon ground nutmeg
½ teaspoon cardamom
⅔ cup (151 grams) Coconut Butter (page 33); if hand mixing, softened, page 137
4 large eggs, at room temperature

Zest of 1 orange
1 tablespoon vanilla
2 green bananas (c. 300 grams)
1 tablespoon apple cider vinegar
½ cup almond butter (page 38)
About 1 cup sweetener to taste (See options on page 18. I especially like part brown sweetener.)
1½ cup nuts, such as walnuts or pecans, soaked and toasted if possible (page 40)

- Preheat the oven to 350°F. Line your pans with parchment paper that hangs over the edge like handles.

- In a food processor or mixing bowl place the almond meal, baking soda, salt, cinnamon, nutmeg, and cardamom. Mix well. Add the coconut butter and mix to a thick paste.

- To the mixture add eggs, zest, vanilla, banana, vinegar, almond butter, and sweetener. Process well until the banana is liquefied.

- Pulse in nuts briefly and pour into the baking pan.

- Bake mini loaves for 20 to 22 minutes, 7 x 3-inch pans for 35 to 45 minutes, 9 x 5-inch pan for 40 to 50 minutes, 9-inch square pan for 25 to 35 minutes.

- Cool in the pans for 1 hour. Chill 1 hour for easy slicing.

Gluten-free	Dairy-free	Egg-free	Meat-free	Tree Nut-free	Vegan	Diabetic-friendly	Candida-friendly	High-protein	10 minutes or less
●	●		●			●	●		

CHOCOLATE PUMPKIN BREAD

If pumpkin bread is good, then chocolate pumpkin bread is much, much better. Rich and full-bodied, the two flavors blend perfectly together. This easy recipe is moist and dense, filled with pure cacao and spices. Since the recipe makes several loaves, you can slice and freeze leftovers for breakfast next week.

YIELD: Three 4.5 x 2.5-inch mini loaves; two 7 x 3-inch loaves; one 9 x 5-inch loaf; or a 9-inch square pan • **EQUIPMENT:** A food processor is helpful but not required

½ cup almond meal

¼ cup pure cacao powder

1 teaspoon baking soda

¼ heaping teaspoon unprocessed salt

1½ tablespoons pumpkin pie spice

½ cup (113 grams) Coconut Butter (page 33); if hand mixing, softened, page 137

3 large eggs (165 grams)

½ cup almond butter (page 38)

Zest of 1 orange

⅔ cup cooked fresh pumpkin or squash pulp, about 165 grams

2 teaspoons vanilla

¼ teaspoon maple flavor

2 teaspoons apple cider vinegar

About 1¼ cups sweetener to taste (See options on page 18. I really like the flavor of part brown sweetener in this.)

1¼ cups nuts, such as walnuts or pecans, soaked and toasted if possible (page 40)

- Preheat the oven to 350°F. Line the baking pan with parchment paper that hangs over the edges like handles.

- In a food processor or mixing bowl, place the almond meal, cacao, baking soda, salt, and spice. Process well. Add the coconut butter, and mix well to a paste.

- To the mixture, add eggs, almond butter, zest, pumpkin, vanilla, maple, vinegar, and sweetener.

- Pulse in the nuts briefly and pour the batter into the lined pan.

- Bake mini loaves for 20 to 22 minutes, 7 x 3-inch pans for 35 to 45 minutes, 9 x 5-inch pan for 40 to 50 minutes, 9-inch square pan for 25 to 35 minutes.

- Cool in the pan for 1 hour. Chill 1 hour for easy slicing.

Gluten-free	Dairy-free	Egg-free	Meat-free	Tree Nut–free	Vegan	Diabetic-friendly	Candida-friendly	High-protein	10 minutes or less
●	●		●			●	●		

CRANBERRY ORANGE CARDAMOM BREAD

This moist cranberry loaf has a rich, buttery flavor with a hint of orange and cardamom, a favorite for the holidays or any time of year. It uses unsweetened cranberries to give your blood sugar a break. Freeze leftovers with wax or parchment paper between slices in an airtight container. Cranberry bread makes a lovely breakfast with Orange Marmalade (page 245) and almond butter (page 38).

YIELD: Three 4.5 x 2.5-inch mini loaves; two 7 x 3-inch loaves; one 9 x 5-inch loaf; or a 9-inch square pan • **EQUIPMENT:** A food processor is helpful but not required

1¾ cups almond meal

½ cup arrowroot flour

1 teaspoon baking soda

½ teaspoon unprocessed salt

1 teaspoon ground cardamom

2 teaspoons nutritional yeast

½ cup (113 grams) Coconut Butter (page 33); if hand mixing, softened, page 137

5 large eggs at room temperature

Zest of 1 orange

Pulp of 1 orange, peeled, sliced, and seeded

2 tablespoons lemon juice

1 teaspoon apple cider vinegar

1 tablespoon vanilla

About ¾ cup sweetener to taste (see options on page 18)

2 cups whole unsweetened cranberries, fresh, or frozen, thawed, and well drained

- Preheat the oven to 350°F. Line the baking pans with parchment paper that hangs over the edges like handles.

- In a food processor or large mixing bowl, place the almond meal, arrowroot, baking soda, salt, cardamom, and nutritional yeast. Mix well. Add the coconut butter and mix to a thick paste.

- Add the eggs, orange zest, orange pulp, lemon juice, vinegar, vanilla, and sweetener. Mix well.

- Pulse in the cranberries briefly so they remain in chunks, not mush. Or chop them coarsely and stir in by hand. Pour into baking pans.

- Bake mini loaves for 20 to 22 minutes, 7 x 3-inch pans for 35 to 45 minutes, 9 x 5-inch pan for 40 to 50 minutes, 9-inch pan for 25 to 35 minutes.

- Cool in the pan for 1 hour. Chill 1 hour for easy slicing.

Gluten-free	Dairy-free	Egg-free	Meat-free	Tree Nut–free	Vegan	Diabetic-friendly	Candida-friendly	High-protein	10 minutes or less
●	●		●			●	●		

LEMON BREAD

Very lemony, very tasty, and so easy to make, this is a moist bread with a pound cake texture that you can serve warm or cold. The recipe uses coconut butter, which gives it an unusually rich flavor and mellow sweetness. Check out the luscious variations below: Lemon Ginger Bread with Basil and Lemon Poppyseed Bread. Try this bread plain or with Blueberry Chia Jam (page 244).

YIELD: Three 4.5 x 2.5-inch mini loaves; or two 7 x 3-inch loaves; or a 9-inch square pan • **EQUIPMENT:** A food processor is helpful but not required

1½ cups almond meal
1 teaspoon baking soda
¼ heaping teaspoon unprocessed salt
2 tablespoons ground white chia seeds (optional)
¾ cup (170 grams) Coconut Butter (page 33); if hand mixing, softened, page 137

5 large eggs at room temperature
Zest of 1 orange (optional) for yellow color
Zest of 1½ lemons
⅓ cup lemon juice
1 teaspoon apple cider vinegar
2 teaspoons vanilla
About 1 cup sweetener to taste (see options on page 18)

- Preheat the oven to 350°F. Line the baking pans with parchment paper that hangs over the edges like handles.
- In a food processor or mixing bowl place the almond meal, baking soda, salt, and chia seeds, if using. Process well. Add the coconut butter and mix well. Add the eggs, orange zest (if using), lemon zest, lemon juice, vinegar, vanilla, and sweetener. Mix well and pour into baking pans.
- Bake mini loaves for 20 to 22 minutes, 7 x 3-inch pan for 35 to 40 minutes, 9-inch square pan for 25 to 35 minutes.
- Cool in the pan for 1 hour. Chill 1 hour for easy slicing.

VARIATIONS:

Lemon Ginger Bread with Basil
Follow the previous recipe. With the sweetener, add 2 inches of fresh ginger root, finely diced. Mix well. Add ¼ cup tightly packed chopped basil and mix very briefly. Pour into baking pans.

Lemon Poppyseed Bread
Follow the previous recipe. With the sweetener, add ½ cup poppyseeds and mix well. Pour into baking pans.

Gluten-free	Dairy-free	Egg-free	Meat-free	Tree Nut-free	Vegan	Diabetic-friendly	Candida-friendly	High-protein	10 minutes or less
●	●		●			●	●		

OLD-WORLD SWEET POTATO BREAD WITH PECANS

This dense and spicy bread will fill your kitchen with a wonderful aroma. It's a moist, rustic loaf with an exquisite flavor of pecans and cinnamon. Use sweet potato cubes that are cooked and well drained. If you're mixing by hand, mash the sweet potato pulp before adding it to the mix. A great use for leftover sweet potatoes, this bread tastes scrumptious plain, with Orange Marmalade (page 245), or with any Homemade Nut Butter (page 38).

YIELD: Three 4.5 x 2.5-inch mini loaves; two 7 x 3-inch loaves; one 9 x 5-inch loaf; or a 9-inch square pan • **EQUIPMENT:** A food processor is helpful but not required

¾ cup almond meal

1 teaspoon baking soda

¼ heaping teaspoon unprocessed salt

2 tablespoons pumpkin pie spice

⅔ cup (151 grams) Coconut Butter (page 33); if hand mixing, softened, page 137

4 large eggs, at room temperature

Zest of 1 orange

1 tablespoon vanilla

¼ teaspoon maple flavor

1 tablespoon apple cider vinegar

2-inch piece fresh ginger root, diced, or ¼ teaspoon ground ginger

1 cup (about 200 grams) sweet potato

About ¾ cup sweetener to taste (See options on page 18. I like part brown sweetener in this recipe.)

1½ cups pecans, soaked and toasted if possible (see page 40)

- Preheat the oven to 350°F. Line the baking pans with parchment paper that hangs over the edges like handles.

- In a mixing bowl or food processor, place the almond meal, baking soda, salt, and spice. Mix well. Add the coconut butter, and mix well again. To the mixture, add the eggs, zest, vanilla, maple, vinegar, ginger, sweet potato, and sweetener and process until smooth.

- Pulse in the pecans briefly and pour the batter into the baking pan.

- Bake mini loaves for 20 to 22 minutes, 7 x 3-inch pans for 35 to 45 minutes, 9 x 5-inch pan for 40 to 50 minutes, 9-inch square pan for 25 to 35 minutes.

- Cool in the pan for 1 hour. Chill 1 hour for easy slicing.

Gluten-free	Dairy-free	Egg-free	Meat-free	Tree Nut–free	Vegan	Diabetic-friendly	Candida-friendly	High-protein	10 minutes or less
●	●		●			●	●		

ZUCCHINI BREAD

This moist, satisfying bread with cinnamon, cardamom, and nuts is completely flourless. Instead of flour, it uses coconut butter and almond meal for a rich, grain-free loaf. You won't notice the zucchini—its mellow pulp melts right into the bread, creating a subtle sweetness and light texture. If batter is too runny, add a bit more almond meal. Easy to bake and freeze, this bread tastes divine with Paleo Cream Cheese (page 43) or Orange Honey Butter (page 251).

YIELD: Three 4.5 x 2.5-inch mini loaves; two 7 x 3-inch loaves; one 9 x 5-inch loaf; or a 9-inch square pan • **EQUIPMENT:** A food processor is helpful but not required

½ cup almond meal
1 teaspoon baking soda
¼ heaping teaspoon unprocessed salt
1½ tablespoons ground cinnamon
¼ teaspoon nutmeg, grated or ground
¼ teaspoon ground cardamom
⅔ cup (151 grams) Coconut Butter (page 33); if hand mixing, softened, page 137
4 large eggs, at room temperature

Zest of 1 orange
1 tablespoon vanilla
1 cup (about 200 grams) grated zucchini
1 tablespoon apple cider vinegar
½ cup almond butter (page 38)
About 1 cup sweetener to taste (See options on page 18. I like part brown sweetener in this recipe.)
1½ cup chopped nuts, soaked and toasted if possible (page 40)

- Preheat the oven to 350°F. Line the baking pans with parchment paper that hangs over the edges like handles.

- In a food processor or mixing bowl, add the almond meal, baking soda, salt, and spices. Process well. Add the coconut butter and mix until it resembles a paste. Add the eggs, zest, vanilla, zucchini, vinegar, almond butter, and sweetener. Mix well.

- Pulse in the nuts briefly and pour the batter into the baking pans.

- Bake mini loaves for 20 to 22 minutes, 7 x 3-inch pans for 35 to 45 minutes, 9 x 5-inch pan for 40 to 50 minutes, 9-inch square pan for 25 to 35 minutes.

- Cool in the pan for 1 hour. Chill for 1 hour for easy slicing.

VARIATION: Chocolate Zucchini Bread
Follow the recipe above with these additions:
  With the dry ingredients add ⅓ cup pure cacao powder.
  Add ½ cup additional sweetener.

Gluten-free	Dairy-free	Egg-free	Meat-free	Tree Nut-free	Vegan	Diabetic-friendly	Candida-friendly	High-protein	10 minutes or less
●	●		●			●	●		

APPLE SPICE MUFFINS, EGG-FREE

Everybody loves these muffins, with the warm flavors of apple, cinnamon, and cloves. The cool thing about them, and what surprises my vegan and egg-free friends, is that there are no eggs in this recipe—none at all. The mixture of apple pulp, chia seeds, and agar powder creates egg-free muffins that rise in the oven and don't fall! These don't rise quite as much as other muffins made with eggs, but you'll forget about that when you taste them! It works best if all the ingredients are at room temperature, and not cold. A batch of twelve muffins can last a long time—freeze them in resealable bags and pull them out to reheat for a quick breakfast treat. Hint: They're even better with Orange Marmalade (page 245).

YIELD: Twelve muffins • **EQUIPMENT:** Food processor

¾ cup plus 2 tablespoons almond meal

2 teaspoons ground cinnamon

¼ teaspoon cloves

¼ teaspoon ginger

½ teaspoon nutmeg

½ teaspoon baking soda

¼ heaping teaspoon unprocessed salt

About ¼ cup sweetener to taste (See options on page 18. Part brown sweetener is especially delicious in this.)

2 Granny Smith apples, cored, in coarse chunks, including peel (about 300 grams)

2 tablespoons whole white chia seeds

1 tablespoon vanilla

1 cup almond butter (page 38)

2 teaspoons apple cider vinegar

Zest of 1 orange (optional)

4 teaspoons agar powder dissolved in ¼ cup boiling water

¾ cup chopped nuts, such as almonds, walnuts, or pecans, soaked and toasted if possible (page 40)

- Preheat the oven to 350°F. Grease a 12-cup muffin tin with coconut oil and dust with coconut flour.

- In a medium mixing bowl, whisk together the dry ingredients: almond meal, cinnamon, cloves, ginger, nutmeg, baking soda, salt, and sweetener.

continues

- In a food processor, add the apple, chia seeds, vanilla, almond butter, vinegar, and zest, if using. Mix well for several minutes. Open the machine, scrape the sides, and continue to mix until liquefied.

- Place the agar powder in a warm mug, as heat helps to activate its thickening power. Stir in ¼ cup boiling water until the agar dissolves. Cover and let it sit for 2 minutes. Then immediately add the dissolved agar to the wet ingredients in the food processor and mix completely.

- Add the dry ingredients to the food processor. Mix well. Add the nuts and pulse in briefly.

- Working quickly, since the rising action is now beginning, spoon the batter into the muffin cups. Bake for 20 to 24 minutes, until a toothpick comes out clean, and muffins are dry enough to lift from the bottom of the cups. Enjoy!

Gluten-free	Dairy-free	Egg-free	Meat-free	Tree Nut-free	Vegan	Diabetic-friendly	Candida-friendly	High-protein	10 minutes or less
●	●	●	●		●	●	●		

BLUEBERRY LEMON MUFFINS

Freshly grated lemon zest makes these muffins extra flavorful. Most blueberry muffins get soggy when the blueberries sink to the bottom. Tip #1: To avoid sinking berry syndrome, freeze your fresh blueberries—just put the package in the freezer for 2 hours. Tip #2: Layer the blueberries with the batter into the muffin tin. If you can't locate fresh blueberries, just use frozen blueberries, unthawed. These muffins taste fantastic with Paleo Butter (page 45) and Blueberry Chia Jam (page 244).

YIELD: Twelve muffins • **EQUIPMENT:** A food processor is helpful but not required

2 cups almond meal
½ teaspoon baking soda
2 tablespoons ground white chia seeds
¼ heaping teaspoon unprocessed salt
1 cup (227 grams) Coconut Butter (page 33); if hand mixing, softened, page 137
5 large eggs at room temperature

Zest of 1 lemon
Zest of 1 orange
⅓ cup lemon juice
2 teaspoons vanilla
About ⅔ cup sweetener to taste (see options on page 18)
6 ounces fresh blueberries, frozen for 2 hours or more

- Preheat the oven to 350°F. Grease a 12-cup muffin tin with coconut oil and dust with coconut flour.

- In a mixing bowl or food processor, place the almond meal, baking soda, chia seeds, and salt. Process well.

- Add the coconut butter and mix well to a thick paste.

- To the mixture, add the eggs, lemon zest, orange zest, lemon juice, vanilla, and sweetener. Process well until completely mixed.

- Pour one-half of the batter into the muffin cups. Sprinkle half of the frozen blueberries into the muffin cups. Then cover them with the remaining batter, and dot the tops with the rest of the berries. It's best to work quickly, because the muffins are rising, and you want to get these babies in the oven. Bake for 22 to 28 minutes, until a toothpick comes out clean. Cool in the pan for 15 minutes.

Gluten-free	Dairy-free	Egg-free	Meat-free	Tree Nut-free	Vegan	Diabetic-friendly	Candida-friendly	High-protein	10 minutes or less
●	●		●			●	●		

CRANBERRY PECAN MUFFINS

This moist, melt-in-your-mouth, muffin is chock full of high-antioxidant cranberries and crunchy pecans. They're unsweetened cranberries, of course, to help keep your blood sugar in balance. Rich coconut butter provides the primary flour in these grain-free muffins. Try these muffins with Orange Marmalade (page 245).

YIELD: Twelve muffins • **EQUIPMENT:** A food processor is helpful but not required

⅔ cup almond meal
½ teaspoon baking soda
¼ teaspoon unprocessed salt
1¼ cups (283 grams) Coconut Butter (page 33); if hand mixing, softened, page 137
Zest of 1 orange
1 teaspoon apple cider vinegar
4 large eggs at room temperature
2 teaspoons vanilla
About 1 cup sweetener to taste (see options on page 18)
1 cup chopped pecans, soaked and toasted if possible (page 40)
1 cup unsweetened whole cranberries, fresh, or frozen, thawed,
    and well drained. Or ½ cup dried unsweetened cranberries.

- Preheat the oven to 350°F. Grease a 12-cup muffin tin with coconut oil and dust with coconut flour.

- In a mixing bowl or food processor, place the almond meal, baking soda, and salt. Add the coconut butter and mix to a thick paste. To the mixture, add the zest, vinegar, eggs, vanilla, and sweetener. Mix well until completely incorporated.

- Pulse in the pecans and cranberries briefly.

- Spoon the batter into the muffin cups. Bake for 22 to 24 minutes, or until a toothpick comes out clean. Cool in the pan for 15 minutes.

Gluten-free	Dairy-free	Egg-free	Meat-free	Tree Nut-free	Vegan	Diabetic-friendly	Candida-friendly	High-protein	10 minutes or less
●	●		●			●	●		

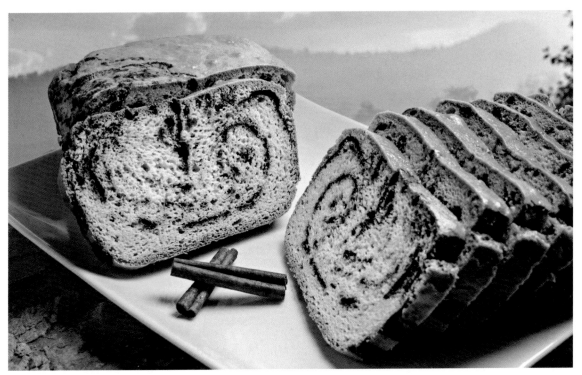

Cinnamon Swirl Bread, page 56

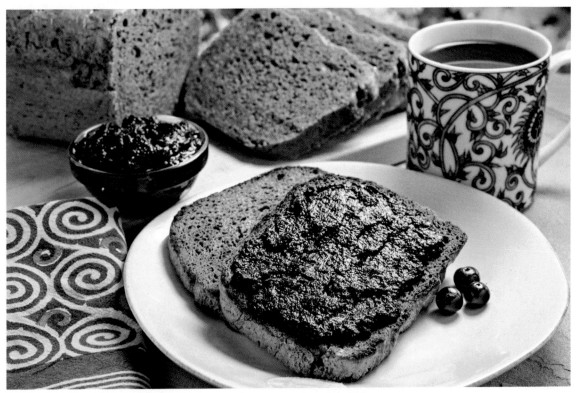

Fluffy Almond Butter Bread, page 54, with Blueberry Chia Jam, page 244

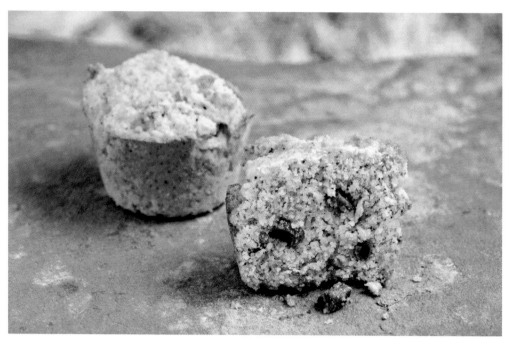

Bacon Chili Cornbread Mini Muffins, page 71

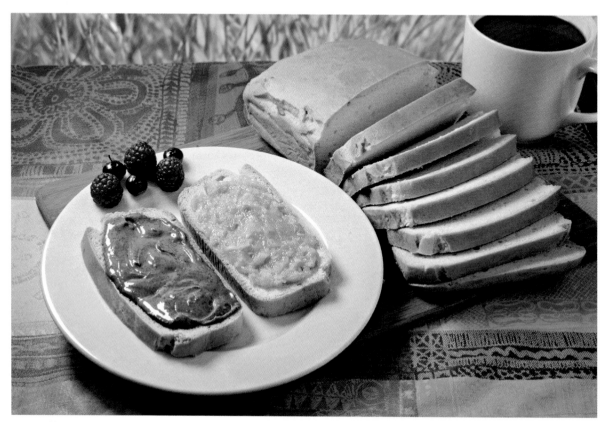

Fluffy White Bread, page 55, with Almond Butter, page 38, and Orange Marmalade, page 245

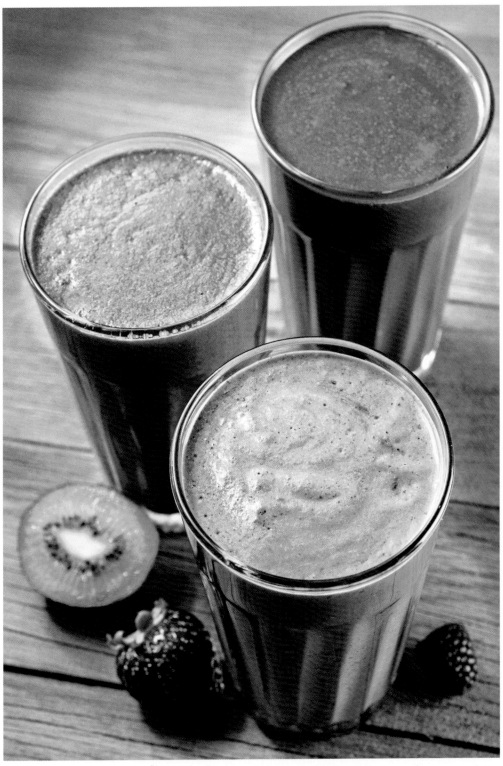

Peaches and Greens Smoothie, page 87, High-Protein Kefir Berry Smoothie, page 85, Chocolate Almond Pick-Me-Up, page 83

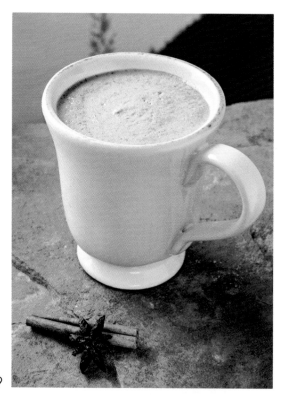

Chai Tea, page 99

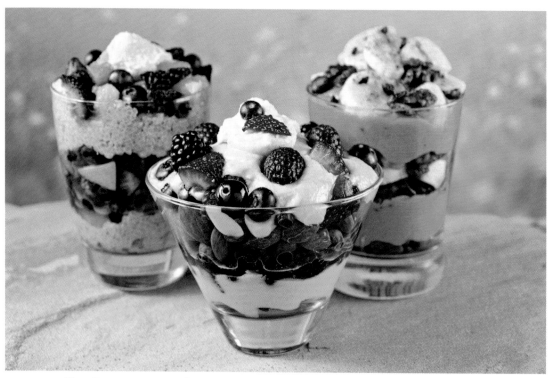

Chia Tapioca Fruit Parfait, page 93, Pumpkin Banana Nut Parfait, page 95,
Lemon Berry Parfait, page 94

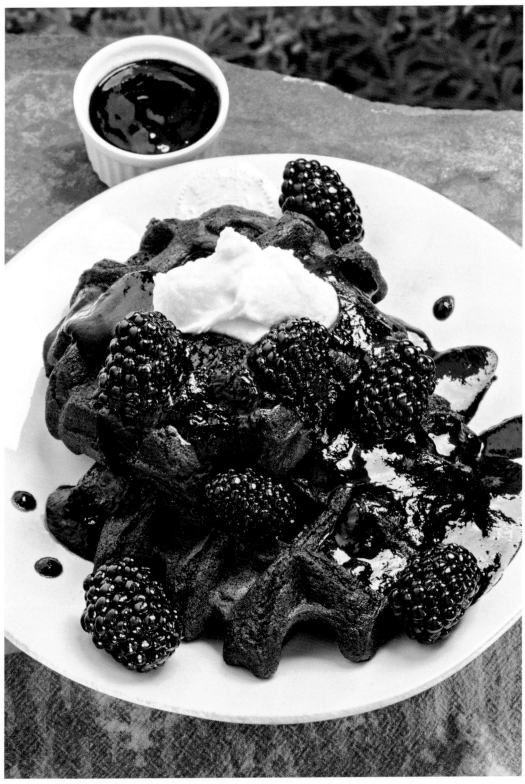

Chocolate Brownie Superfood Waffles, page 125, with Blackberry Sauce, page 243

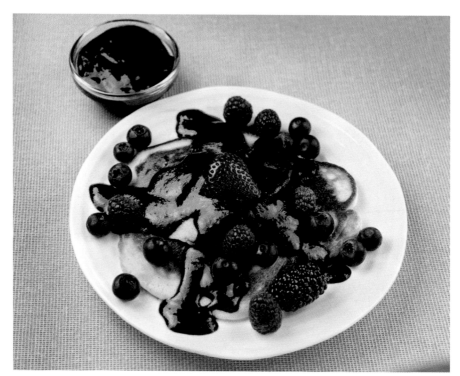

Blueberry Pancakes, page 117, with Berrylicious Sauce, page 243

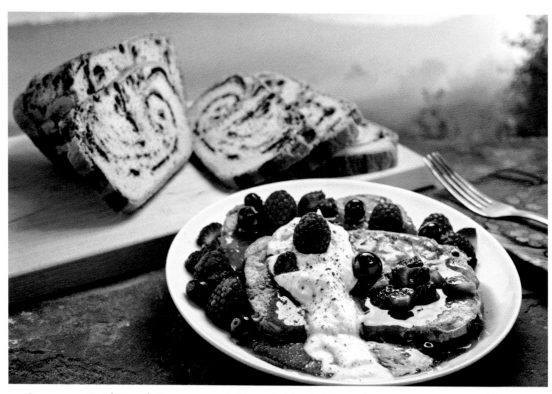

Cinnamon Swirl French Toast, page 131, with Maple Flavor Syrup, page 246, and berries

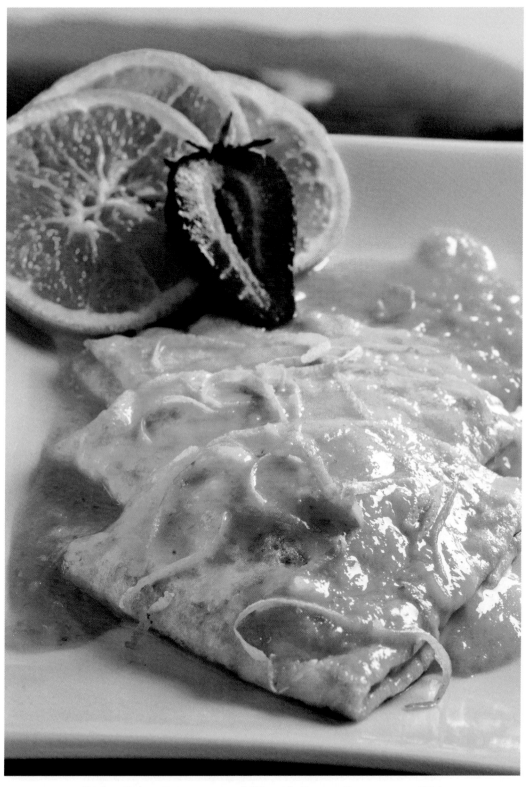

Perfect Paleo Crepes, page 133, with Suzette Sauce, page 134

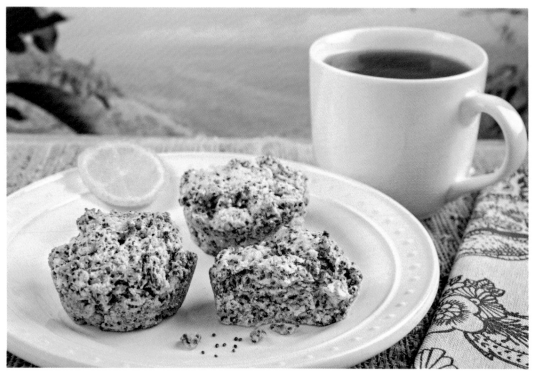

Lemon Chia Seed Muffins, Egg-Free, page 149

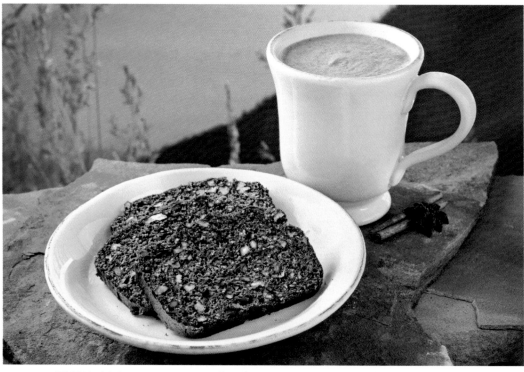

Old-World Sweet Potato Bread with Pecans, page 143, Chai Tea, page 99

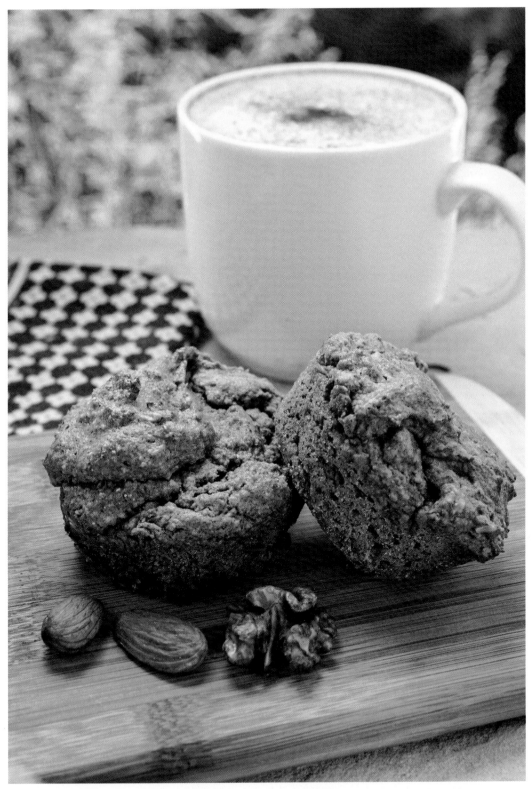

Apple Spice Muffins, Egg-Free, page 145, with Cappuccino, page 98

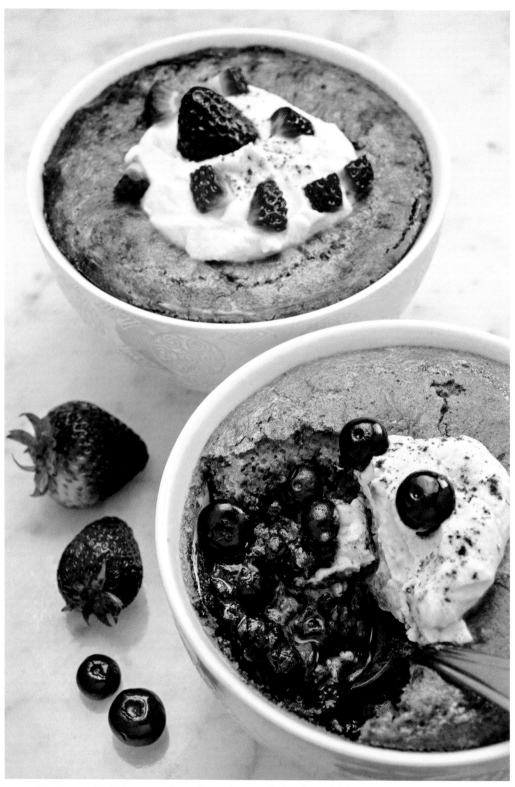

Blueberry Cobbler in a Cup, Strawberry Rhubarb Cobbler in a Cup, page 166

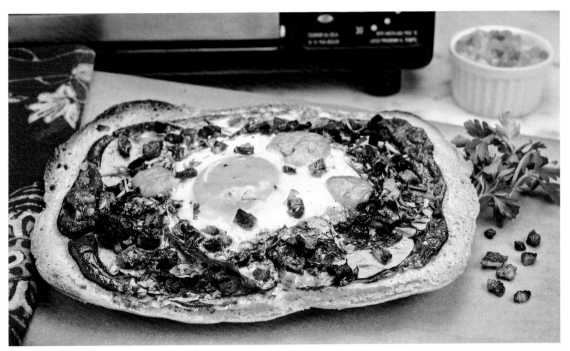

Personal Pizza for One, page 180, with Homemade Bacon Bits, page 42,
and Spicy Cheese Sauce, page 258

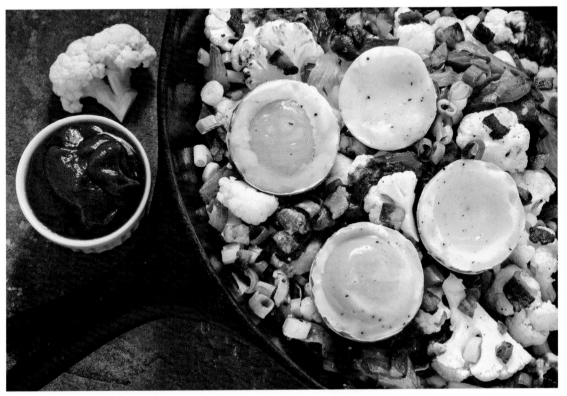

Bacon Cauliflower Hash with Eggs, page 171, and Homemade Ketchup, page 255

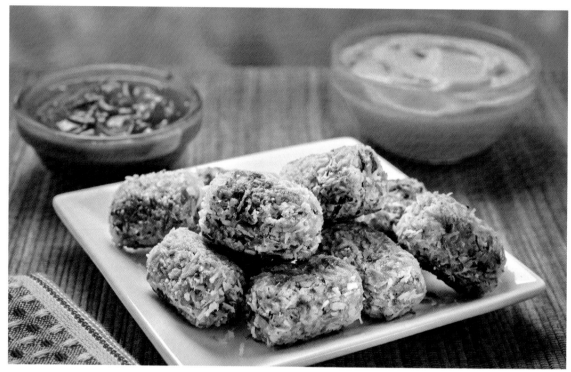

Sweet Potato Tots, page 185, with Homemade Ketchup, page 255,
and Spicy Cheese Sauce, page 258

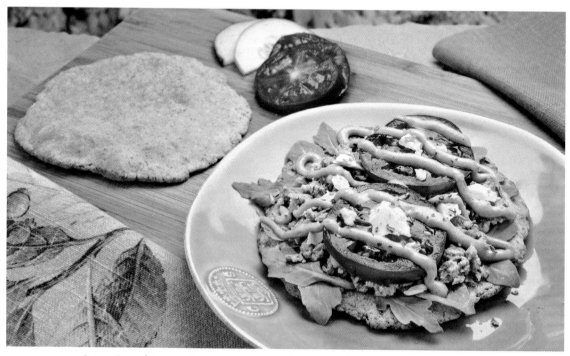

Open-Faced Focaccia, page 179, with Zesty Italian Sausage, page 239,
arugula, and Parmesan Cheese Sauce, page 257

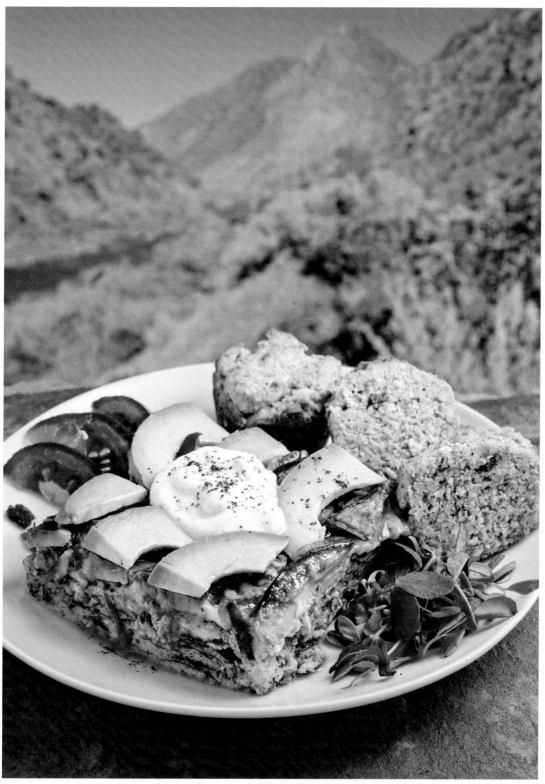
Cowboy Baked Eggs, page 203, with Bacon Chili Cornbread, page 71

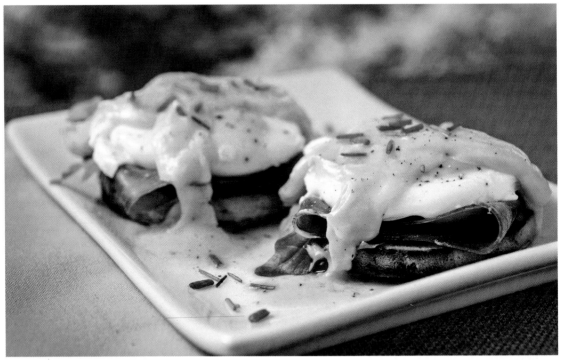

Eggs Benedict, page 208, on English Muffins, page 67, with Hollandaise Sauce, page 254

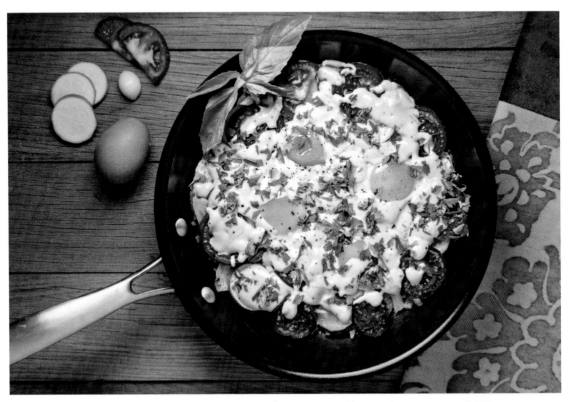

Italian Baked Eggs, page 204, with Parmesan Cheese Sauce, page 257

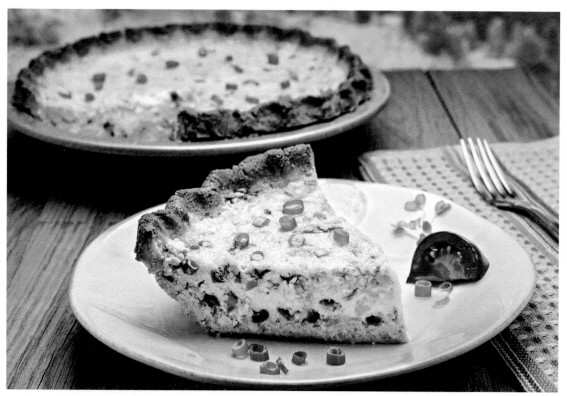

Quiche Lorraine, page 222

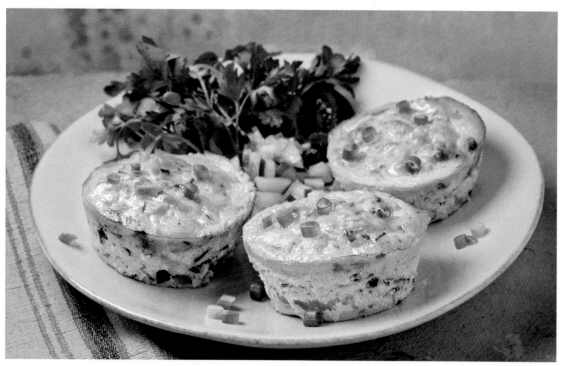

Wild Salmon Leek Mini Quiches, page 225

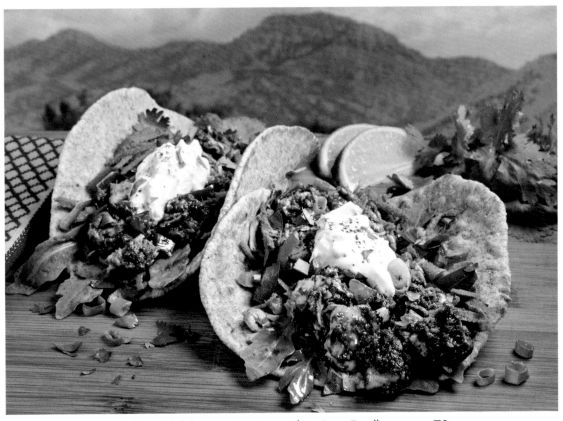

Chicken Adobo, page 229, on Chia Corn Tortillas, page 73

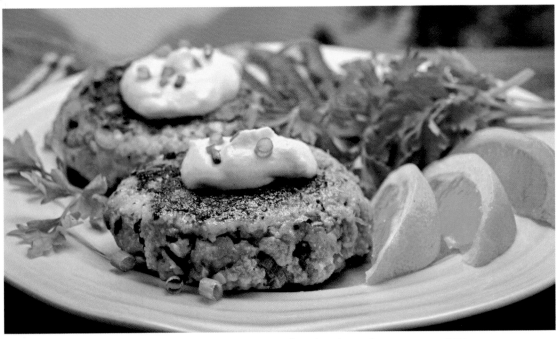

Wild Salmon Cakes, page 233, with Paleo Sour Cream, page 256

LEMON CHIA SEED MUFFINS, EGG-FREE

I love the fresh taste of lemon poppy seed muffins. This totally unique recipe uses chia seeds, apple, and agar powder rather than poppy seeds and eggs. Agar powder is a tasteless seaweed—dissolve it in boiling water and it thickens much like albumen in egg. The result is a completely egg-free muffin that actually rises in the oven. Chia seeds give you an extra benefit of protein-packed, high omega-3 nutrition. Follow the recipe closely—it works—even though they don't rise quite as high as gluten flours. It works best if all the ingredients are at room temperature, and not cold. Wrap and freeze leftovers for a quick, nutritious breakfast.

YIELD: Twelve muffins • **EQUIPMENT:** Food processor

⅔ cup almond meal
½ teaspoon baking soda
¼ teaspoon unprocessed salt
About ¾ cup sweetener to taste (see options on page 18)
1 Granny Smith apple in coarse chunks, including peel (160 grams)
2 teaspoons vanilla

¾ cup (170 grams) Coconut Butter (page 33)
Zest of 1 lemon
⅓ cup lemon juice
1 teaspoon apple cider vinegar
½ cup whole black chia seeds
4 teaspoons agar powder dissolved in ¼ cup boiling water

- Preheat the oven to 350°F. Grease a 12-cup muffin pan with coconut oil and dust with coconut flour.

- In a medium mixing bowl, whisk together the almond meal, baking soda, salt, and sweetener. Set aside.

- In a food processor, add the apple, vanilla, coconut butter, zest, lemon juice, vinegar, and chia seeds. Mix well until apple is liquefied. Open the machine, scrape the sides, and mix again.

- Place agar powder in a warmed mug, as heat helps to activate its thickening power. Stir in ¼ cup boiling water until agar dissolves. Cover and let it sit for 2 minutes—you can set a timer. Immediately add hot agar to the food processor and mix well.

- Add the dry ingredients to the wet ingredients in the food processor. Mix well until all the ingredients are incorporated. Spoon the batter into muffin cups. Bake for 20 to 24 minutes, until a toothpick comes out clean, the muffins are baked on the bottom and loosening from the cups. Enjoy!

Gluten-free	Dairy-free	Egg-free	Meat-free	Tree Nut-free	Vegan	Diabetic-friendly	Candida-friendly	High-protein	10 minutes or less
●	●	●	●		●	●	●		

PUMPKIN MUFFINS WITH STREUSEL TOPPING

These flavorful muffins are a great use for leftover pumpkin. And here's a shortcut—when you don't have cooked pumpkin on hand, it's a snap to use squash, which is easier to peel and steam. Save even more time when you buy precubed squash. Coconut butter and almond butter together create a rich, moist texture. Fresh ginger and orange zest add a pleasant zing. Use fresh pumpkin or squash that's cooked and well drained. Canned pumpkin will be too liquid. I find it easiest to grind all the nuts (1½ cups total) first. Be sure to press the streusel topping into the muffins a bit with your fingers before baking, so it stays on the muffins.

YIELD: Twelve muffins • **EQUIPMENT:** A food processor is helpful but not required

STREUSEL TOPPING:
- ¾ cup chopped nuts, such as walnuts or pecans, soaked and toasted if possible (page 40)
- 1 tablespoon coconut oil, melted
- 2 tablespoons almond meal
- ¼ teaspoon ground cinnamon
- A pinch of unprocessed salt
- About 2 tablespoons sweetener to taste (see options on page 18)

MUFFINS:
- ¾ cup almond meal
- 1 teaspoon baking soda
- ¼ heaping teaspoon unprocessed salt
- 2 tablespoons pumpkin pie spice
- ½ cup (113 grams) Coconut Butter (page 33); if hand mixing, softened, page 137
- 4 large eggs
- ½ cup almond butter
- Zest of 1 orange
- ¾ cup (200 grams) cooked fresh pumpkin or precubed squash (if mixing by hand, mashed)
- 2-inch piece of fresh ginger root, peeled and chopped, or ¼ teaspoon ground ginger
- 1 tablespoon vanilla
- ¼ teaspoon maple flavor
- 1 tablespoon apple cider vinegar
- About 1 cup sweetener to taste (see options on page 18)
- ¾ cups chopped nuts, such as almonds, walnuts, or pecans, soaked and toasted if possible (page 40)

continues

continued

- Preheat the oven to 350°F. Grease and flour a 12-cup muffin tin with coconut oil and coconut flour.

- Mix the streusel topping in a small bowl. Combine all the ingredients, stir until crumbly, and set aside.

- In a food processor or mixing bowl, place the almond meal, baking soda, salt, and spice. Process well. Add the coconut butter and mix to a thick paste. Add the eggs, almond butter, zest, pumpkin, ginger, vanilla, maple, vinegar, and sweetener. Process well. Pulse in the nuts briefly and spoon into muffin cups. Top with the streusel topping and press it in lightly with your fingers.

- Bake for 17 to 22 minutes, or until a toothpick inserted comes out clean.

Gluten-free	Dairy-free	Egg-free	Meat-free	Tree Nut-free	Vegan	Diabetic-friendly	Candida-friendly	High-protein	10 minutes or less
●	●		●			●	●		

CINNAMON APPLE SOUR CREAM COFFEECAKE MUFFINS

This recipe tastes just like my mom's coffeecake. It's a fluffy muffin with a chunky apple filling and cinnamon streusel topping. Just before baking, the apple cinnamon filling is briefly mixed into the cake batter for a marbled effect. These muffins are super-easy to save for a grab-and-go breakfast another day. Just freeze them in a BPA-free storage container. Or if you'd like a traditional round coffeecake, follow the variation below. This recipe tastes absolutely scrumptious with Hot Caramel Sauce (page 248).

YIELD: Twelve coffeecake muffins; serves six • **EQUIPMENT:** A food processor is helpful but not required

STREUSEL TOPPING:
¾ cup chopped nuts, such as almonds or pecans, soaked and toasted if possible (page 40)

1 tablespoon coconut oil, melted

1 tablespoon brown sweetener (see options on page 18)

1 tablespoon almond meal

¼ teaspoon ground cinnamon

A pinch of unprocessed salt

APPLE CINNAMON FILLING:
1½ Granny Smith apples (about 240 grams) cored and chopped in ¼ inch pieces, including the peel

1 tablespoon lemon juice

About 6 tablespoons brown sweetener (see options on page 18)

2 tablespoons ground cinnamon

1 teaspoon cardamom

¼ heaping teaspoon cloves

Zest of 1 orange

2 tablespoons coconut oil, melted

CAKE BATTER:
1⅔ cups almond meal

½ teaspoon baking soda

½ teaspoon unprocessed salt

1½ tablespoons nutritional yeast

⅓ cup (75 grams) Coconut Butter (page 33); if hand mixing, softened, page 137

4 large eggs at room temperature

½ teaspoon apple cider vinegar

2 teaspoons vanilla

About ½ cup sweetener to taste (see options on page 18)

continues

continued

- Preheat the oven to 350F°. Grease a 12-cup muffin pan with coconut oil, and dust with coconut flour.

- Mix the streusel topping in a small bowl. Combine all the ingredients and stir until crumbly; set aside.

- For the apple cinnamon filling: In a large mixing bowl, combine all the ingredients. Mix well to coat the apples and set aside in the bowl.

- For the batter: In a food processor or medium mixing bowl, add the almond meal, baking soda, salt, and nutritional yeast. Mix well. Add the coconut butter and mix to a thick paste. To this mixture, add the eggs, vinegar, vanilla, and sweetener. Mix well.

- Now put this batter into the apple mixture. Stir gently with a rubber spatula in five to eight circular motions for a marbled effect. Do not mix completely. You want each muffin to get a taste of each. Spoon the two-color batter into the muffin cups.

- Sprinkle the muffins with streusel topping and press it in lightly with your fingers.

- Bake for 20 to 25 minutes, or until the toothpick comes out clean.

VARIATION: Cinnamon Apple Sour Cream Coffeecake
Here's my mom's traditional coffeecake—except it's Paleo, of course. Line a 9-inch springform or cake pan with a circle of parchment paper. Follow the recipe above. Pour the marbled batter into the pan. Bake for 20 to 25 minutes. Cool for 15 minutes, cut into wedges, and serve.

Gluten-free	Dairy-free	Egg-free	Meat-free	Tree Nut-free	Vegan	Diabetic-friendly	Candida-friendly	High-protein	10 minutes or less
●	●		●			●	●		

7

BARS, CRUMBLES, AND OTHER SWEETS

"Lead me not into temptation;
I can find the way myself."
—Rita Mae Brown

This chapter transforms your most decadent sweets into miraculously nutrient-dense breakfasts. They do a double duty, which is critical at the start of your day. That is, they offer on the one hand a delicious sweet starter, and on the other hand a guarantee of stable metabolism and balanced blood sugar all day.

It's all about sugars, carbs, and proteins. Everyone knows that a breakfast high in carbs and sugars causes a temporary blood sugar rush in the body. Eventually when the blood sugar falls, the drop can make you feel frustrated and irritable later in the day, not to mention hungry and craving more sweets. Your sugar crash could hit at the worst possible moment. A daily sugar roller coaster over a long period of time takes a lasting toll on your health.

These recipes are the best of both worlds: decadent sweets that are truly healthy and nutritious. When you eliminate the sugars, carbs, and refined ingredients, and substitute hunt-and-gather ingredients, you can reinvent any treat in a healthy form.

Here's a great example: I ran a nutritional analysis to compare two breakfast cookies. #1 is a popular conventional cookie. #2 is the Big Breakfast Cookie on page 157. Both of these cookies weigh the same. Cookie #1 is made of wheat flour, butter, honey, eggs, rolled oats, coconut, and dried fruits. Cookie # 2 is made of Granny Smith apple,

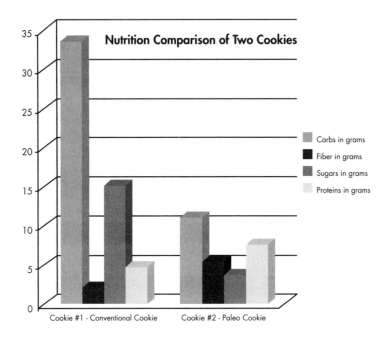

Nutrition Comparison of Two Cookies

Carbs in grams
Fiber in grams
Sugars in grams
Proteins in grams

Cookie #1 - Conventional Cookie   Cookie #2 - Paleo Cookie

green banana, eggs, nuts, chia seeds, coconut, cacao nibs, and chicory root sweetener. They're both super-crunchy and delicious. Guess which one will be the most powerful fuel for your day?

Here are the surprising results. The conventional breakfast cookie is extremely high in carbs and sugars, low in fiber and protein. That's a recipe for a sugar rush and a crash following. In contrast, Cookie #2, the Paleo Big Breakfast Cookie, is very low in carbs and sugars. It has more than double the fiber and almost twice as much protein as the conventional cookie.

My Paleo cookie will build strong body tissues. It will hold you for many hours. Even better, it's free of refined ingredients. This is great news for all cookie monsters!

You can compute your own nutritional analysis free online. While these recipes may seem like decadent desserts, they are healthy breakfasts made from the highest order of foods known to Nature. They contain the best nutrient-dense ingredients and superfoods available, to bring the benefits of the ancestral diet right into your modern kitchen.

————

BIG BREAKFAST COOKIES

High in protein, loaded with nutrition, these scrumptious crunchy cookies are a great grab-and-go breakfast. Green banana is low in sugars and carbs and high in resistant starch, which helps cultivate healthy intestinal flora. These cookies freeze well in a simple freezing container. They'll reward you with delicious quick breakfasts and snacks anytime.

YIELD: Twenty large cookies • **EQUIPMENT:** A food processor or blender is helpful but not required

1 Granny Smith apple, in coarse chunks with peel (if mixing by hand, grated)
1 green banana (if mixing by hand, mashed)
1 cup roasted almond butter (page 38)
2 large eggs
2 tablespoons chia seeds, white or black
⅓ cup coconut oil
1 tablespoon vanilla
¼ teaspoon maple flavor
1½ cups shredded unsweetened coconut

⅔ cup almond meal
¾ teaspoon unprocessed salt
2 tablespoons ground cinnamon
About ⅔ cup sweetener to taste (see options on page 18)
3 cups whole toasted nuts, such as pecans, almonds, walnuts, pumpkin seeds, sunflower seeds, soaked and toasted if possible (page 40)
¼ cup unsweetened cacao nibs (optional)

- Preheat the oven to 350°F. Cover the baking sheets with parchment paper.

- In a food processor or blender, place the apple, green banana, almond butter, eggs, chia seeds, oil, vanilla, and maple. Process well until liquefied. Add the shredded coconut and process again to grind it as much as possible.

- In a large mixing bowl, whisk together the almond meal, salt, cinnamon, and sweetener. Add in the nuts and cacao nibs, if using.

- Pour the processor liquid contents into the mixing bowl and mix with a spatula into a thick batter. Use a ¼-cup measure or an ice-cream scoop to drop mounds of dough on each of two baking sheets. Flatten and shape the cookies with greased hands or a spatula into flat rounds about ½ inch thick.

- Bake for 20 to 25 minutes until the underside is golden brown.

Gluten-free	Dairy-free	Egg-free	Meat-free	Tree Nut-free	Vegan	Diabetic-friendly	Candida-friendly	High-protein	10 minutes or less
●	●		●			●	●	●	

BLUEBERRY CRUMBLE BARS

I'm always looking for easy, nutrient-dense breakfasts that are high in protein and low in sugar—and these bars, with their rich blueberry filling, fit the bill! They're loaded with antioxidants, omega-3s, and protein. And they're egg-free. I like to assemble this dish the night before and bake it in the morning. You can wrap these bars individually and freeze them for a quick breakfast later.

YIELD: Sixteen bars • **EQUIPMENT:** Food processor

CRUST:
2 tablespoons ground white chia seeds soaked 15 minutes in 6 tablespoons filtered water
½ cup almond meal
About ⅓ cup sweetener to taste (see options on page 18)
1 teaspoon vanilla
½ teaspoon unprocessed salt
¼ cup almond butter (page 38)
1 tablespoon of your favorite protein powder (optional)
1 cup shredded unsweetened coconut

FILLING:
10 ounces (1 cup) blueberries, fresh, or frozen, thawed, and well drained
1 avocado, pitted and peeled
1 tablespoon arrowroot flour
1 teaspoon lemon zest
2 tablespoons lemon or lime juice
1 teaspoon vanilla
1 teaspoon ground cinnamon
2 pinches cloves
2 pinches nutmeg
About ⅔ cup sweetener to taste (see options on page 18)

TOPPING:
½ cup shredded unsweetened coconut
⅓ cup chopped nuts, such as almonds, pecans, or walnuts, soaked and toasted if possible (page 40)

- Preheat the oven to 350°F. Cover a 9-inch square baking pan with parchment paper.

- Crust: In a food processor, combine the soaked chia seeds, almond meal, sweetener, vanilla, salt, almond butter, and protein powder, if using. Mix well.

- Pulse in the coconut briefly so it remains in large pieces. The crust will be quite thick.

continues

continued

- Press the crust evenly into the bottom of the pan. Bake for 10 minutes and remove from the oven.

- For the filling, to the empty food processor add all the filling ingredients. Process until well blended. The filling will be thick and puddinglike.

- Spread the filling evenly over the crust. Sprinkle the coconut and nuts on top. Press them in with your fingers.

- Bake for 25 to 30 minutes or until the center is set.

- Cool for 15 minutes. Cut into bars and enjoy!

Gluten-free	Dairy-free	Egg-free	Meat-free	Tree Nut–free	Vegan	Diabetic-friendly	Candida-friendly	High-protein	10 minutes or less
●	●	●	●		●	●	●	●	

CARAMEL CHOCOLATE SUPERFOOD BARS

With a chocolate brownie on the bottom and a crisp pecan topping, this might seem to be the most decadent recipe in the book. However—surprise! It's also the most nutrient-dense food in the book. A perfect way to start a high-energy day, these bars are packed with nutrition from protein powder, vegetables, apple, chia seeds, and your favorite superfoods. So as your taste buds are spinning with joy, your whole body is relaxing and saying thanks! Wrap them individually—they freeze beautifully for up to 3 months. This makes a large 9 x 13-inch pan so you can enjoy them for a while.

YIELD: Thirty-six to forty bars • **EQUIPMENT:** A food processor is helpful but not required

BROWNIE BASE:
1 cup almond meal
½ cup (113 grams) Coconut Butter (page 33); if mixing by hand, soften butter by placing the container in a bowl of warm water
½ cup pure cacao powder
½ teaspoon unprocessed salt
½ apple, cored, cut in chunks with the peel (if mixing by hand, grate the apple)
2 tablespoons coconut oil
½ cup almond butter
4 large eggs
1 tablespoon vanilla
Zest of 1 orange
1 cup sweet potato or pumpkin pulp (if mixing by hand, cooked and mashed)
1 tablespoon chia seeds
About 1 cup sweetener to taste (See options on page 18. This recipe is quite delicious with half brown sweetener.)

OPTIONAL SUPERFOODS IN THE BROWNIE:
1 scoop of your favorite protein powder
1 small scoop of your favorite green powder
1 tablespoon nutritional yeast
1 tablespoon presoaked hiziki or wakame seaweed
1 tablespoon maca powder
1 teaspoon bee pollen
1 dropper of ChlorOxygen
A handful of baby spinach

PECAN PIE TOPPING:
¼ cup warm water
2 large eggs
2 teaspoons vanilla
½ teaspoon apple cider vinegar
¼ teaspoon maple flavor
¼ cup melted coconut oil
About 1½ cups sweetener to taste (See options on page 18. Half brown sweetener is especially delicious in this recipe.)
¼ heaping teaspoon salt
2½ cups pecans, soaked and toasted if possible (page 40)

continues

continued

- Preheat the oven to 350°F. Line a 9 x 13-inch pan with parchment paper that hangs over the edge like handles.

- For the brownie base, in a food processor or mixing bowl, place all the brownie ingredients and mix well.

- Add your favorite superfoods and mix again until all the ingredients are combined. The batter should be quite thick.

- Pour into the baking pan.

- For the topping, in the same food processor or bowl, place the water, eggs, vanilla, vinegar, maple, coconut oil, sweetener, and salt. Mix well until all the ingredients are combined.

- Pulse in the pecans briefly, so they're slightly chopped. The topping should be like a thick frosting.

- Drop the pecan pie topping in spoonfuls over the brownie batter in the pan, and spread smooth.

- Bake for 30 to 35 minutes, or until a toothpick comes out clean.

- Cool or chill and cut into bars.

Gluten-free	Dairy-free	Egg-free	Meat-free	Tree Nut-free	Vegan	Diabetic-friendly	Candida-friendly	High-protein	10 minutes or less
●	●		●			●		●	

APPLE BREAD PUDDING

Filled with rich cinnamon and apple, this is a whole new concept in decadent bread pudding. That's because it's super-easy to make, low in carbs, and healthy! It's a great way to use any leftover grain-free bread and is especially yummy made with Fluffy White Bread (page 55) or Cinnamon Swirl Bread (page 56). Oh, please try it with Maple Pecan Syrup (page 246)! You can put it together in the evening and bake it in the morning. Or defrost the bread overnight, assemble, and bake in the morning. Freeze for up to 6 weeks in squares individually wrapped, in a freezing container.

YIELD: One 9-inch square pan; serves four

5 cups grain-free bread cut in
 ½-inch cubes

1 apple, chopped fine, including peel

4 large eggs

3 cups unsweetened full-fat coconut milk
 (page 13)

2 teaspoons ground cinnamon

¼ teaspoon nutmeg

¼ teaspoon allspice

1 tablespoon lemon juice

Zest of 1 orange

Pulp of 1 orange, peeled, sliced, and seeded;
 if mixing by hand, chopped

1 tablespoon vanilla

½ teaspoon maple flavor

About 1 cup sweetener to taste
 (See options on page 18. I especially like
 half brown sweetener here.)

- Preheat the oven to 350°F. Grease a 9-inch square pan. Put bread cubes and chopped apple into the pan and mix it around briefly to combine.

- In any blender, food processor, or mixing bowl, add the eggs, coconut milk, cinnamon, nutmeg, allspice, lemon juice, orange zest, orange pulp, vanilla, maple, and sweetener. Mix until well combined. Pour the mixture over the bread and push it down with a spatula so the bread is completely covered. You can allow it to soak for an hour or overnight. Or, you can skip soaking and bake now.

- Bake for about 45 minutes, or until the top springs back when lightly tapped. Serve with your favorite sauce.

Gluten-free	Dairy-free	Egg-free	Meat-free	Tree Nut–free	Vegan	Diabetic-friendly	Candida-friendly	High-protein	10 minutes or less
●	●		●	●		●	●		

APPLE BERRY CRISP

While crisps are often dessert territory, this easy recipe makes for a wonderful breakfast with its hints of berries, orange, and nutmeg. Organic apples are best: you don't have to peel them, and the peels are chock full of nutrients. If you choose to use peeled apples, the crisp will be a bit softer. Serve warm or at room temperature with Coconut Cream Topping (page 249). Freeze leftovers in a BPA-free container for future breakfasts.

YIELD: One 9-inch square pan; serves four

5 to 6 Granny Smith apples
1 tablespoon lemon juice
About 2 tablespoons sweetener to taste
  (See options on page 18. Brown
  sweetener is quite delicious here.)
1½ teaspoons ground cinnamon
¼ teaspoon nutmeg
Zest of ½ orange
½ cup unsweetened berries, fresh
  or frozen, such as raspberries,
  cranberries, or strawberries

STREUSEL TOPPING:
1 cup shredded unsweetened coconut
1 teaspoon ground cinnamon
About 1 tablespoon sweetener
  (see options on page 18)
¼ teaspoon unprocessed salt
2 tablespoons melted coconut oil
  (put the jar in a bowl of warm water)
¼ cup chopped nuts, such as almonds or
  walnuts, soaked and toasted if possible
  (page 40)

- Preheat the oven to 375°F. Grease a 9-inch square pan.

- Core the apples and slice them very thin into a large mixing bowl (peeling them is optional). Sprinkle with lemon juice, sweetener, cinnamon, nutmeg, and orange zest. Add the berries and stir the mixture gently. Sweeten to taste depending on the tartness of your berries.

- Put the apples and berries into the baking dish. They'll be very tall, but don't worry, they'll cook down.

- For the streusel topping, in a small mixing bowl, mix the coconut, cinnamon, sweetener, salt, coconut oil, and chopped nuts. Sprinkle this mixture over the apples and press it in.

- Bake for 35 to 40 minutes, until the apples and peels are soft.

Gluten-free	Dairy-free	Egg-free	Meat-free	Tree Nut–free	Vegan	Diabetic-friendly	Candida-friendly	High-protein	10 minutes or less
●	●	●	●		●	●	●		

PEAR GINGER CRISP WITH BERRIES

The luscious aroma of pears and cinnamon will pull anyone out of bed. High-antioxidant berries—your choice—add flavor and nutrition. Organic pears are best: you don't have to peel them, and the peels are loaded with nutrients. If you choose to use peeled pears, the crisp will be a bit softer. This crisp can be assembled in the evening and baked in the morning. Serve plain or with Coconut Cream Topping (page 249). Freeze leftovers in a BPA-free container for future breakfasts.

YIELD: One 9-inch square pan; serves four

4 pears sliced very thinly (⅛ inch), including the peel

1 cup unsweetened raspberries, blueberries, or cranberries

1 teaspoon ground cinnamon

2 tablespoons arrowroot flour

2 tablespoons grated fresh ginger or ½ teaspoon ground

Zest of 1 orange

About 2 tablespoons sweetener to taste (see options on page 18)

STREUSEL TOPPING:

1 cup pecans, finely chopped

1 tablespoon coconut oil, melted (place the jar in a bowl of warm water)

About 2 tablespoons sweetener to taste (see options on page 18)

3 tablespoons shredded coconut

¼ teaspoon ground cinnamon

¼ teaspoon unprocessed salt

- Preheat the oven to 350°F. Place the pear slices and berries in the bottom of a greased 9-inch square baking pan.

- In a mixing bowl, whisk together the cinnamon, arrowroot, ginger, zest, and sweetener. Sprinkle over the pears and stir the mixture in. Press the fruit flat.

- For the topping, in a small bowl, stir together with a fork the pecans, coconut oil, sweetener, coconut, cinnamon, and salt. Sprinkle over the fruit and poke holes in the top with a sharp tool so the flavors mix in baking.

- Bake for 30 minutes until the pears are tender and the topping is golden brown.

Gluten-free	Dairy-free	Egg-free	Meat-free	Tree Nut–free	Vegan	Diabetic-friendly	Candida-friendly	High-protein	10 minutes or less
●	●	●	●		●	●	●		

PEACH SHORTBREAD CRUMBLE

This easy crumble is a favorite breakfast when peaches are in season—and when they're not I just use frozen peaches. A hint of cardamom and citrus zest give it a delicate, exquisite flavor. Oh, and the individual pieces freeze well for another fantastic breakfast, so try not to eat the whole pan.

YIELD: One 9-inch square pan, about sixteen pieces • **EQUIPMENT:** A food processor is helpful but not required

2 cups almond meal
¼ teaspoon salt
¼ teaspoon ground cardamom
⅛ teaspoon ground cinnamon
⅛ teaspoon grated nutmeg
¾ cup (170 grams) Coconut Butter (page 33); if mixing by hand, soften butter by placing the container in a bowl of warm water
2 large eggs
Zest of 1 orange
1 teaspoon vanilla
About ½ cup or a little more sweetener to taste (see options on page 18)
2 peaches, fresh or frozen, sliced very thinly (⅛ inch)

- Preheat the oven to 350°F. Grease a 9-inch square inch pan and dust with coconut flour.

- In a medium bowl or food processor, mix the almond meal, salt, cardamom, cinnamon, and nutmeg. Add the coconut butter and mix to a thick paste. Add the eggs, zest, and vanilla and mix until well combined. Sweeten to taste. Mix well until a crumbly mixture forms.

- Pat three-quarters of the mixture into the baking pan, pressing firmly. Layer the peach slices on top. Scatter the remaining crumbs over the peaches.

- Bake for 30 minutes, until the top is slightly brown. Cool for 30 minutes, and cut into squares.

Gluten-free	Dairy-free	Egg-free	Meat-free	Tree Nut-free	Vegan	Diabetic-friendly	Candida-friendly	High-protein	10 minutes or less
●	●		●			●	●		

BLUEBERRY COBBLER IN A CUP

High in protein, and low in carbs, this "cup cake" makes an easy breakfast for one. Just whisk together the batter when you wake up, and bake. By the time you're dressed and checking your messages, breakfast is served. Enjoy it plain or with Coconut Cream Topping (page 249), if desired.

YIELD: One 12-ounce cobbler

FRUIT BASE:
1 cup blueberries, fresh or frozen, thawed, and well drained
½ teaspoon lemon juice
¼ teaspoon ground cinnamon
2 to 3 tablespoons chopped nuts, such as almonds or walnuts, soaked and toasted if possible (page 40)
Sweetener is optional, 0 to 2 tablespoons (see options on page 18)

BATTER:
1 large egg
2 tablespoons unsweetened coconut milk (page 35), almond milk (page 36), or filtered water
1 tablespoon olive oil or melted coconut oil
A dash of vanilla
¼ teaspoon ground cinnamon
A pinch of unprocessed salt
⅓ cup almond meal
⅛ teaspoon baking soda
About 2 tablespoons sweetener to taste (See options on page 18. Half brown sweetener is quite delicious in this recipe.)

- Preheat the oven to 350°F. Get out a 12-ounce, ovenproof cup, cereal bowl, or ramekin. Put the blueberries, lemon juice, cinnamon, nuts, and sweetener in the cup. Stir well and press into the bottom of the cup.

- In a separate small bowl, whisk together the egg, milk, olive oil, vanilla, cinnamon, salt, almond meal, baking soda, and sweetener.

- Pour the batter over the fruit in the cup.

- Bake on a baking tray for 18 to 25 minutes. Cool and enjoy!

VARIATION: Strawberry Rhubarb Cobbler in a Cup
Follow the recipe above, replacing the blueberries with ½ cup sliced strawberries and ½ cup diced rhubarb.

Gluten-free	Dairy-free	Egg-free	Meat-free	Tree Nut–free	Vegan	Diabetic-friendly	Candida-friendly	High-protein	10 minutes or less
●	●		●			●	●		

SWEET POTATO POPOVERS

One of my greatest delights as a child was eating Dad's popovers straight out of the oven. With their hot, light, and hollow inside, these delectable treats will melt in your mouth. The #1 secret: Do not open the oven. It's so much fun to watch through the glass oven door as these babies literally pop over the muffin cups. A nutritious, high-protein breakfast, sweet potatoes add healthy fiber, vitamin B$_6$, and beta-carotene. These are easy to make in the blender. To make light popovers, your batter needs to be fairly thin and liquidy. So I suggest using coconut milk that's not very thick. If you're using thick coconut milk, thin it with filtered water. These taste incredulicious with Paleo Butter (page 45) or Orange Honey Butter (page 251).

YIELD: Twelve popovers • **EQUIPMENT:** Any blender or food processor

4 large eggs
1 cup unsweetened coconut milk (page 35) or almond milk (page 36);
   if it is thick, use ½ cup milk, ½ cup filtered water
3 tablespoons coconut oil
1 cup arrowroot flour
½ teaspoon ground cinnamon
½ teaspoon unprocessed salt
½ sweet potato, raw or cooked, in ½-inch cubes
   (about 100 grams or ⅔ cup pulp)

Have all the ingredients at room temperature, especially the eggs and milk.

- Preheat the oven to 425°F. Grease a 12-cup muffin tin very well with coconut oil and dust with coconut flour. Place the muffin tin on top of the stove to warm while you're making the batter.

- In any blender or food processor, add the eggs, milk, coconut oil, arrowroot, cinnamon, salt, and sweet potato. Blend well until smooth and the sweet potato is completely liquefied. The batter will be quite thin.

- Pour the batter into the muffin cups two-thirds to three-quarters full. Bake for 15 minutes without opening the oven. Set the timer and DO NOT PEEK. After 15 minutes turn the oven temperature down to 375°F. Set the timer, and bake for another 15 minutes again. Do not open the oven, just watch them through the window! Then reduce the temperature to 325°F and bake for another 10 minutes. Set the timer.

continues

- Open the oven and quickly use a sharp knife to make a small slit in the top of each popover to allow steam to escape. This helps them bake in the center, which keeps the shape stable. Then close the oven and bake for another 10 minutes.

- Remove the popovers from the oven and allow them to cool on a rack for 1 to 2 minutes. Then remove them with a knife gently around the edges. Serve warm.

Gluten-free	Dairy-free	Egg-free	Meat-free	Tree Nut–free	Vegan	Diabetic-friendly	Candida-friendly	High-protein	10 minutes or less
●	●		●	●		●	●		

8

MY DAD'S
FAVORITE HEARTY BREAKFASTS

"Food should make you healthy!"
—Robb Wolf

My dad's breakfasts were always astonishing. He was an early riser, and my sisters and I were often lured out of sleep by tantalizing smells wafting through the house. Weekends were his time to perform in the kitchen, and we enjoyed every bite. We downed savory East Indian wraps filled with curried lentils, root vegetables cooked every way imaginable, homemade lamb patties, Mexican turtle soup, Asian stir-fries, and countless other breakfasts from around the world.

Hash with fried potatoes was always a breakfast favorite and a great way to use leftovers and a variety of veggies. But Paleo hash browns without potatoes?

Now that my diet is Paleo, I've discovered so many new ways to make hash.

Sweet potato hash is a staple favorite. Cauliflower makes a satisfying hash, as you'll find in Bacon Cauliflower Hash with Eggs (page 171) and Wild Salmon Cauliflower Hash (page 174). For flexibility, I offer a recipe for Design Your Own Hash Browns (page 173), where you can choose your root vegetable from squash, sweet potato, turnip, rutabaga, celeriac, or yam. These recipes are truly Paleo, even though you may be hunting and gathering in your own kitchen.

I hope you enjoy this potpourri of flavors inspired by my dad. He taught me that when we really decide to make something healthy and delicious, we somehow find a way to rethink and revise our old ways of doing things—including breakfast.

169

SWEET POTATO HASH WITH TURKEY APPLE SAUSAGE

This hearty breakfast is almost too easy to write down. I'm including it because sweet potatoes topped with fried eggs are incredibly delicious, and they make an ideal substitute for white potatoes, which aren't Paleo. I'm betting there won't be leftovers. But if there are, freeze them for up to 6 weeks in a BPA-free container. When you want to use them, defrost in the refrigerator overnight, and reheat in a pan for a quick breakfast. Serve with Homemade Ketchup (page 255).

YIELD: Serves four

2 large sweet potatoes
12 ounces bulk Turkey Sausage with Apple and Sage (page 238), or your favorite sausage
2 cloves garlic, diced
1 large yellow onion, sliced
½ large red onion, sliced
5 green onions, diced

½ red bell pepper, sliced
½ teaspoon ground cumin
¼ teaspoon smoked paprika
4 eggs
1 teaspoon coconut oil
Unprocessed salt and black pepper to taste

- Peel the sweet potatoes and slice into ½-inch cubes.

- Add the sweet potato cubes to a medium pot with 1 inch of filtered, salted water. Bring to a boil and then turn down to a very low simmer to steam until almost cooked—al dente—for 5 to 10 minutes. Then drain with a colander or strainer and set aside.

- In a large nonstick skillet, brown the sausage over medium heat until almost cooked.

- To the skillet add the garlic, yellow and red onion, green onions, bell pepper, cumin, and smoked paprika. Cook until almost soft, about 5 minutes. Add the sweet potatoes and cook for 5 minutes more.

- Meanwhile, fry your eggs. Heat the coconut oil in another large skillet over medium heat. When a drop of water sizzles, it's ready. Break the eggs one at a time onto the hot skillet. Turn the heat down and cook for 1 to 3 minutes, until they are done as you like them.

- Season your hash to taste with salt and pepper. Serve with a fried egg on top.

Tip: To slice the sweet potatoes, it's quickest to slice them crossways first. Then pile the slices face-up and slice them vertically and horizontally into cubes

Gluten-free	Dairy-free	Egg-free	Meat-free	Tree Nut-free	Vegan	Diabetic-friendly	Candida-friendly	High-protein	10 minutes or less
●	●			●		●	●	●	

BACON CAULIFLOWER HASH WITH EGGS

While you may think of potatoes when you think of breakfast hash, this quick and easy comfort breakfast uses cauliflower rather than fried potatoes—with yummy, healthy results. Prepare your eggs any way you like them. You can soft boil them as in the photo in the insert. Or you can fry them over easy or sunny-side up, or scramble or poach them. This recipe is very flexible, so go ahead and use your favorite ingredients. Homemade Bacon Bits (page 42) make it super-easy—look for sugar-free non-GMO bacon. Freeze leftover hash for up to 6 weeks in BPA-free containers for a quick breakfast when you need it.

YIELD: Serves four, with one egg each

4 large eggs
3 tablespoons coconut or olive oil
3 cloves garlic, diced
1 large onion, preferably red, sliced
Unprocessed salt and pepper to taste
1½ cups raw sweet potato, in bite-size pieces
1 large head raw cauliflower, cut into bite-size florets
4 green onions, sliced
½ cup Homemade Bacon Bits (page 42), or sliced bacon,
    cooked and diced (optional)

- Decide how you would like your eggs cooked. If you're doing soft-boiled eggs, start them now—in 6 minutes both the eggs and hash will be ready. If you're frying, poaching, or scrambling the eggs, do that as the hash is finishing.

- To make soft-boiled eggs, fill a medium saucepan half-full with water. Bring it to a boil and turn the heat down to medium. Using a large spoon, carefully lower the eggs one at a time into the boiling water. Set the timer for 6 minutes.

- For the hash: In a large skillet, melt the oil over medium high heat. Add the garlic and sauté very briefly, for 1 minute. Add the onion, salt, and pepper. Sauté for 2 minutes, until the onions begin to soften.

- Add the sweet potato and sauté for 2 minutes. Add the cauliflower. Sauté for 3 to 5 minutes, stirring gently. Add green onions and Homemade Bacon Bits. Cover the pan and cook for 1 to 2 minutes, stirring occasionally and adjusting the heat so it doesn't burn. When the cauliflower is barely al dente, the hash is done. Cover and remove from the heat.

continues

continued

- If you're frying, scrambling, or poaching the eggs, do this now. To open soft-boiled eggs, immerse them in cold water so they stop cooking. Use a table knife to cut an opening around the middle of each egg. Give the shell a light whack with the knife and lift off the top half of the egg. Serve eggs in the half-shell, or use a teaspoon to scoop it out into the hash. Serve the hash with the eggs on top.

Gluten-free	Dairy-free	Egg-free	Meat-free	Tree Nut-free	Vegan	Diabetic-friendly	Candida-friendly	High-protein	10 minutes or less
●	●			●		●	●	●	

DESIGN YOUR OWN HASH BROWNS

Hash is a super-flexible recipe—you can choose your own root vegetable, greens, and the meat is optional. (Woo hoo! A chance to clean out the fridge.) Any hash needs a dollop of Homemade Ketchup (page 255).

YIELD: Serves two hungry persons or four light eaters • **EQUIPMENT:** There are several ways to grate the root vegetable: (1) Grate with a box grater, (2) Use the grating blade of a food processor, (3) Use a mandoline slicer, or (4) Use a julienne peeler.

6 ounces meat, such as natural bacon, ham, or sausage, diced (non-GMO and
　　sugar-free if possible; meat is optional)
2 cloves garlic, minced
1 red onion, sliced
2 cups coarsely grated root vegetable, such as squash, sweet potato, turnip,
　　rutabaga, celeriac, or yams (about ½ pound)
Unprocessed salt and pepper to taste
⅓ cup filtered water or Homemade Bone Broth (page 47)
2 green onions, sliced
2 cups coarsely chopped greens, such as kale, spinach, chard, dandelion greens,
　　arugula, or bok choy
2 to 4 large eggs

- In a large skillet over medium heat sauté the meat for about 2 minutes, if using. Add the garlic and onion, and sauté until the meat is mostly cooked, about 3 minutes.

- Add the grated root vegetable, salt, pepper, and water. Cover the pan to allow the root vegetable to steam cook for 1 minute. Then add the green onions and greens. Cover the pan and steam until the greens begin to soften, for about 2 minutes.

- Make two to four small wells in the veggies in the pan and crack an egg into each well. Cover and steam until the eggs are cooked, adding a tablespoon or two of water (or broth) to the pan to keep the bottom from sticking and to steam the eggs. If you like your yolks runny, 2 minutes should do it. If you like the yolks solid, steam it for 4 to 5 minutes. Serve in the pan.

Gluten-free	Dairy-free	Egg-free	Meat-free	Tree Nut–free	Vegan	Diabetic-friendly	Candida-friendly	High-protein	10 minutes or less
●	●			●		●	●	●	

WILD SALMON CAULIFLOWER HASH

I love this savory hash for its luscious contrast of textures—crispy cauliflower and tender, moist salmon. It's very quick to make and a great use for leftover salmon. You can add a fried egg on top for a crowning touch, although it's just as good without. Freeze leftovers up to 6 weeks in a BPA-free container for a quick breakfast next week. Serve with Paleo Sour Cream (page 256), Homemade Ketchup (page 255), or Hollandaise Sauce (page 254).

YIELD: Serves two

½ pound wild salmon fillet
2 tablespoons coconut oil
1 clove garlic, chopped
1 red onion, sliced
½ cauliflower, in coarse florets
Unprocessed salt and pepper to taste
2 green onions, diced
1 red pepper, in strips
1 teaspoon ground mustard
2 tablespoons lemon juice
2 tablespoons chopped herbs, such as thyme, parsley, cilantro, or basil
2 large eggs (optional)

- To cook the salmon, place the fillet in a small skillet over medium heat with ¼ inch of filtered water. Bring to a boil, cover, and turn down to a very low simmer for about 4 minutes to steam. When it is lighter in color and barely cooked, cool, remove skin and bones, and cut into ½-inch cubes.

- In a skillet, melt the oil over medium-high heat. Sauté the garlic and red onion for 2 minutes until they begin to soften.

- Add the cauliflower, salt, and pepper to taste. Sauté for 3 to 5 minutes, stirring gently to avoid breaking the florets. Stir in the green onions, red pepper, mustard, lemon juice, and herbs. Add the salmon, cover, and cook for a minute or two, stirring occasionally. Adjust the heat so it doesn't burn on the bottom, and add a bit of water if the pan looks dry. When the cauliflower is "al dente" and just barely soft enough to chew, remove from the heat.

continues

continued

- If serving with eggs, heat the coconut oil in another large skillet over medium heat. When a drop of water sizzles, it's ready. Break the eggs one at a time onto the hot skillet. Turn the heat down and cook for 1 to 3 minutes, until they are done as you like them.

- Serve the hash in the pan, topped with fried eggs, if desired.

VARIATIONS:

Serve on a bed of raw spinach or arugula.

Instead of salmon, make it with cooked corned beef, bacon, or ham. Follow the instructions above, except omit the salmon. While the vegetables are cooking, add the meat.

Gluten-free	Dairy-free	Egg-free	Meat-free	Tree Nut–free	Vegan	Diabetic-friendly	Candida-friendly	High-protein	10 minutes or less
●	●			●		●	●	●	

BISCUITS AND GRAVY

Creamy sausage gravy over hot baking powder biscuits is a classic Southern breakfast. It's quick to make in just 15 minutes and will stick to your ribs all morning. Both biscuits and gravy have super-flexible premake options. You can freeze leftovers separately, defrost in the refrigerator overnight, and reheat for a super-quick breakfast next week.

YIELD: Nine 2-inch biscuits with sausage gravy for four

1 recipe Baking Powder Biscuits (page 68)
1 pound bulk Homemade Breakfast Sausage (page 235)
½ onion, chopped
2 tablespoons arrowroot flour
¼ teaspoon ground nutmeg
½ teaspoon sage or poultry seasoning, or 1 tablespoon chopped herbs
   (parsley, thyme, basil)
½ teaspoon nutritional yeast (optional)
1¾ cups unsweetened, full-fat coconut milk (page 13)
Unprocessed salt and black pepper to taste

- Prepare the Baking Powder Biscuits; set aside.

- For the gravy: In a large skillet over medium heat, brown the sausage for 3 minutes. Add the onion and sauté until it begins to soften. Add the arrowroot, nutmeg, sage, and nutritional yeast, if using. Stir to coat the sausage evenly.

- Add the coconut milk and heat just to boiling. Then turn the heat off to not overcook the milk. Adjust salt and pepper to taste. Serve immediately over the biscuits.

Gluten-free	Dairy-free	Egg-free	Meat-free	Tree Nut-free	Vegan	Diabetic-friendly	Candida-friendly	High-protein	10 minutes or less
●	●					●	●	●	

BREAKFAST BURRITOS

One of our favorite grab-and-go Mexican meals, burritos can be personalized to suit everyone's tastes. Whether you prefer avocado or chicken, eggs or salsa, these basic homemade burritos can be varied a thousand ways. I like to spread them with Cilantro Pesto (page 253) or Paleo Sour Cream (page 256). If you can make the wraps ahead and freeze, this is one of the easiest breakfasts in town.

YIELD: Serves two

1 recipe Easy Burrito Wraps (page 76)
1 avocado, pitted, peeled, and mashed
2 teaspoons lemon or lime juice
Unprocessed salt and black pepper to taste
¾ cup cooked meat, such as diced chicken, sautéed beef slices, or sausage
2 large eggs, scrambled
½ cup tomato salsa
⅓ cup chopped cilantro

• Make the Easy Burrito Wraps.

• In a small bowl, stir together the avocado, lemon juice, salt, and pepper.

• Spread it on each wrap.

• Add the meat, eggs, salsa, and cilantro on top.

• Fold in the bottom third of the wrap. Roll it horizontally. Secure it with a toothpick. If you are taking it with you, wrap it in parchment paper or wax paper with tape.

BURRITO VARIATIONS:
Fill them with Scrambled Eggs with Cheese (page 213), Refried Sweet Potatoes (see Huevos Rancheros, page 209), Spicy Chorizo (page 237), or Beef Fajitas with Spicy Cheese Sauce (page 228). Let your imagination go wild.

Gluten-free	Dairy-free	Egg-free	Meat-free	Tree Nut-free	Vegan	Diabetic-friendly	Candida-friendly	High-protein	10 minutes or less
●	●			●		●	●	●	

BREAKFAST TACOS

¡Ay, caramba! When my friends tasted these Paleo tacos, they couldn't believe they contain no corn or cheese. They're so flavorful you'll want to eat several. So this recipe makes four tacos for two. If you can make the tortillas and Spicy Cheese Sauce (page 258) ahead, this breakfast is a snap—just pull them from your stash in the freezer. This is a basic vegetarian taco—the sausage is optional.

YIELD: Four tacos • **EQUIPMENT:** Any blender (for the sauces)

4 Chia Corn Tortillas (page 73) or Plantain Tortillas (page 75)
¼ cup of your favorite tomato salsa
2 to 4 tablespoons Spicy Cheese Sauce (page 258)
2 tablespoons Paleo Sour Cream (page 256), optional

TACO FILLINGS:
6 ounces sausage, such as Spicy Chorizo (page 237) or
   Green Chile Lamb Sausage (page 236) (optional)
4 large eggs, beaten
Unprocessed salt and pepper to taste
A handful of fresh spinach or baby arugula
½ carrot, coarsely grated
A handful of chopped cilantro

- Prepare the tortillas; cover and keep them warm in the oven.

- In a large skillet, brown the sausage, if using. Add the eggs, salt, and pepper, and scramble them together.

- Lay the four tortillas on serving plates. Add the fillings: spinach, grated carrot, sausage and eggs, and chopped cilantro. Top with salsa, Spicy Cheese Sauce, and Paleo Sour Cream, if desired.

Gluten-free	Dairy-free	Egg-free	Meat-free	Tree Nut-free	Vegan	Diabetic-friendly	Candida-friendly	High-protein	10 minutes or less
●	●			●		●	●	●	

OPEN-FACED FOCACCIA WITH SAUSAGE

This recipe is a wonderful Mediterranean-style breakfast, with all the trimmings—see photo in the insert. It's like a taco piled up with goodies that you can eat with your hands. Super-quick and full of flavor, it's the easiest breakfast in town if you make the flat bread, cheeses, and sausage ahead. Just pull them out of the freezer, heat, and enjoy.

YIELD: Serves two • **EQUIPMENT:** Any blender (to make the Parmesan Cheese Sauce and Feta Cheese)

2 pieces Focaccia Flat Bread, Egg-Free (page 77)
3 ounces Zesty Italian Sausage (page 239)
4 ounces baby arugula
6 cherry tomatoes, or one ripe tomato, sliced
1 recipe Parmesan Cheese Sauce (page 257)
2 tablespoons Paleo Feta Cheese (page 44)
2 tablespoons diced herbs, such as oregano or basil

- Warm the focaccia briefly in the oven or a toaster oven.

- In a small sauté pan over medium heat, cook the sausage for about 5 minutes, until done.

- To assemble, put two pieces of focaccia on serving plates. Place the arugula on the focaccia. Put the sausage on top of the arugula. Top with tomatoes, Parmesan Cheese Sauce, Paleo Feta Cheese, and diced herbs.

Gluten-free	Dairy-free	Egg-free	Meat-free	Tree Nut-free	Vegan	Diabetic-friendly	Candida-friendly	High-protein	10 minutes or less
●	●	●				●	●	●	

PERSONAL PIZZA FOR ONE

This breakfast pizza is so simple: you can bake it in a toaster oven and eat it in just a few minutes. The delicious secret is a super-easy crust. If your egg is a nonstandard size, you may need to adjust the batter. To thicken, add a bit more almond meal. To thin it, add a bit of water. I like to top it with Avocado Pesto (page 252), Spicy Cheese Sauce (page 258), spinach, and egg. You can use any sauce or toppings you like. See the photo in the insert.

YIELD: Serves one • **EQUIPMENT:** A toaster oven or an oven with broiler

PIZZA CRUST:
¼ cup almond meal
3 tablespoons arrowroot flour
⅛ teaspoon unprocessed salt
⅛ teaspoon baking soda
1 large egg (55 grams)
2 teaspoons olive oil

OPTIONAL TOPPINGS:
3 tablespoons sauce, such as Avocado Pesto (page 252), Spicy Cheese Sauce (page 258), or your favorite pizza sauce
A handful of arugula or baby spinach
2 tablespoons meat, such as Homemade Bacon Bits (page 42)
2 tablespoons chopped herbs, such as green onions, parsley, cilantro, or oregano
1 large egg
Unprocessed salt and pepper to taste

- Prepare your toppings. Turn a toaster oven to "toast," or preheat oven to broil (500°F). Cover a baking tray with lightly oiled parchment paper about 8 x 6 inches.

- In a cup, whisk together all the ingredients for the crust. The dough should be fairly runny. Pour the batter on the parchment paper and spread it thin. Bake for 3 to 4 minutes, until the top is dry to the touch and you can pick it up.

- Remove the tray from the oven. Flip the bread over onto the tray. Spread it with sauce and your favorite toppings. If preparing with an egg on top, make a well in the center of the veggies, with edges that can hold the runny egg white. This is the tricky part, as there needs to be a barrier of veggies around the egg to keep it on the pizza. Break an egg into the hole. Add salt and pepper.

- Bake again for 3 to 6 minutes, keeping an eye on it. If you like your yolks runny it will take about 3 minutes. If you like the yolks cooked through it will be a bit longer. Remove from the oven and enjoy.

Gluten-free	Dairy-free	Egg-free	Meat-free	Tree Nut-free	Vegan	Diabetic-friendly	Candida-friendly	High-protein	10 minutes or less
●	●					●	●	●	

QUESADILLAS

These quesadillas are like a tortilla sandwich with scrambled eggs and a rich mushroom cheese filling. They're even tastier with a dollop of Paleo Sour Cream (page 256). The tortillas can be made ahead and frozen. Pull them out in the morning for quick breakfast prep.

YIELD: Serves two

1 recipe Easy Burrito Wraps (page 76), Plantain Tortillas (page 75), or Chia Corn Tortillas (page 73)

QUESADILLA FILLING:
1 tablespoon olive or coconut oil
1 clove garlic, crushed
½ cup sliced shiitake mushrooms
2 green onions, sliced
3 large eggs, beaten
2 tablespoons lemon juice
2 tablespoons nutritional yeast

¼ teaspoon salt
Plenty of black pepper
1 tablespoon olive oil
¼ teaspoon chili powder

OPTIONAL INGREDIENTS:
¼ cup cooked chicken pieces
A handful of diced tomatoes
A handful of Homemade Bacon Bits (page 42)
1 tablespoon chopped cilantro
Paleo Sour Cream (page 256)

- Prepare the tortillas, cover, and set aside.

- Heat the oil in a large skillet over medium heat. Add the garlic and mushrooms. Sauté for a few minutes until they start to soften. Add the green onions and any other optional ingredients you like, and sauté briefly.

- Add the eggs and stir to scramble, about 2 minutes.

- In a small cup, stir together the lemon juice, nutritional yeast, salt, pepper, olive oil, and chili powder. Pour over the eggs as they're cooking and stir it in a bit, cooking for 1 minute. Then put the mixture on a plate and set aside.

- To assemble the quesadillas, clean and dry the skillet. Add a bit of oil over medium heat. Put one of the tortillas into the pan. Spoon in some of the mushroom filling, depending how many you're making, and spread it flat. Put another tortilla on top and press it down like a sandwich. No need to flip it—when it's heated through just slip it onto a serving plate and cut into six to eight wedges. Repeat for the next tortillas until the filling is used up.

Gluten-free	Dairy-free	Egg-free	Meat-free	Tree Nut-free	Vegan	Diabetic-friendly	Candida-friendly	High-protein	10 minutes or less
●	●			●		●	●	●	

SOUTHWEST VEGETABLE FRITTERS

These yummy fritters are guaranteed to get anyone to eat their vegetables. Crisp and flavorful, they make an easy breakfast on their own, or serve them with a side of eggs. Freeze leftover fritters first on a baking tray, and then put in a ziplock bag for up to 3 months. Defrost them in the refrigerator overnight for a quick and tasty breakfast. Serve with Cilantro Pesto (page 253), Avocado Pesto (page 252), Paleo Sour Cream (page 256), or your favorite salsa.

YIELD: Six 2½-inch patties

2 large eggs
2 tablespoons onion flakes
1 tablespoon lemon juice
2 tablespoons (28 grams) Coconut Butter (page 33), or any nut butter (page 38)
1 tablespoon nutritional yeast
3 tablespoons fresh cilantro, chopped
¼ teaspoon unprocessed salt

Black pepper to taste
½ cup almond meal, or ⅓ cup coconut flour
½ teaspoon ground cumin
¼ teaspoon chili powder
1 small zucchini, coarsely grated
1 carrot, coarsely grated
2 green onions, chopped
2 tablespoons coconut oil for cooking

- In a medium mixing bowl, beat the eggs. Add the onion flakes, lemon juice, coconut butter, nutritional yeast, cilantro, salt, pepper, almond meal, cumin, and chili powder, if using. Stir to combine. Add the grated vegetables and onions and mix well. The batter will be quite thick.

- In a large nonstick skillet over medium heat, melt the coconut oil. When a drop of water flicked on the surface sizzles, it's ready. Measure ¼ cup of the batter and form six patties in your hands.

- Cook the patties for about 4 minutes on each side or until golden brown. Enjoy.

Gluten-free	Dairy-free	Egg-free	Meat-free	Tree Nut-free	Vegan	Diabetic-friendly	Candida-friendly	High-protein	10 minutes or less
●	●		●	●		●	●		

SPICY SOUTHWEST BREAKFAST POCKETS

A flavorful meal or healthy snack on the go, these zesty Paleo pockets are gluten-free and grain-free. Even better, they freeze beautifully—just pull them out 20 minutes before you need them and heat them in any oven, even a toaster oven, for a quick, satisfying breakfast. These pockets taste delightful with Paleo Sour Cream (page 256). If your eggs are not standard 55 grams each, your dough may be too thick or too runny. If your eggs are smaller, your dough will be thicker. If your eggs are jumbo, the dough will be too runny. To resolve this you can either weigh the eggs or adjust the other ingredients—see instructions below. Freeze pockets up to 3 months in a BPA-free freezing container.

YIELD: Eight to ten pockets

FILLING:
- 2 tablespoons coconut or olive oil
- ½ onion, sliced
- 1 clove garlic, diced
- 4 ounces Homemade Breakfast Sausage (page 235), or your favorite sausage
- ½ teaspoon ground cumin
- ¼ teaspoon ground mustard
- ¼ teaspoon chili powder (optional)
- 1 carrot, coarsely grated or diced
- 2 green onions, diced
- 1 cup fresh greens, such as spinach, arugula, chard, or kale, coarsely chopped
- 1 tablespoon nutritional yeast
- 1 tablespoon lemon juice
- 2 tablespoons cilantro, diced

DOUGH:
- 1 cup almond meal
- ½ cup arrowroot flour
- ½ teaspoon unprocessed salt
- 2 large eggs (110 grams)
- ⅔ cup (151 grams) Coconut Butter (page 33); if mixing by hand, soften butter by placing the container in a bowl of warm water
- 1 tablespoon apple cider vinegar
- 1 tablespoon water, or several tablespoons almond meal, if necessary to adjust consistency of dough before rolling
- Coconut flour, for dusting

- For the filling, in a large skillet over medium heat, place the oil. Sauté the onion and garlic briefly, for about 2 minutes. Add the sausage, cumin, mustard, and chili powder, if using. Sauté until the sausage is almost cooked, about 3 minutes. Add the carrot, green onion, fresh greens, nutritional yeast, lemon juice, and cilantro. Stir together and sauté briefly until the greens are almost wilted, but not yet cooked, for about 2 minutes. Then remove from the heat and set the filling aside.

continues

- Preheat the oven to 350°F. Cover two baking trays with parchment paper.

- For the dough, in a mixing bowl or food processor, place the almond meal, arrowroot, and salt and mix well.

- Add the eggs, coconut butter, and vinegar. Process until it forms a firm dough. If the dough is too thin to roll, mix in almond meal or arrowroot a tablespoon at a time. If it is too thick, add a bit of water a teaspoon at a time. Wrap the dough in parchment paper and press flat. Chill for 15 minutes.

- Form the dough into a ball and place on a counter top lightly dusted with coconut flour. I find it easiest to divide the dough in half to roll and cut. Roll between two layers of parchment or wax paper to ⅛ inch thick. Peel off the top layer of paper. You can use any round object such as an inverted bowl or a pan lid to measure. Cut the dough in 5-inch circles and put each circle on the baking sheet.

- To assemble, place a few tablespoons of filling into half of the dough circle. Fold the other half over and crimp the very edges with a fork. Repeat for all the pockets. Prick a few tiny steam holes in the top with the tip of a knife.

- Brush with olive oil and bake for 15 to 20 minutes, depending on the size of your pockets. Finish them to a beautiful golden brown by turning the oven up to broil for the last few minutes. Just watch carefully and remove them as they begin to brown.

Gluten-free	Dairy-free	Egg-free	Meat-free	Tree Nut-free	Vegan	Diabetic-friendly	Candida-friendly	High-protein	10 minutes or less
●	●					●	●	●	

SWEET POTATO TOTS

Here's an easy, nutrient-rich alternative to traditional white tater tots that everyone loves. These Paleo tots are crispy, flavorful, and packed with beta-carotene and vitamins A and C. Serve with Spicy Cheese Sauce (page 258) or Homemade Ketchup (page 255). You could freeze leftovers up to 3 months in an air-tight container. But alas, there will never be any leftovers—they'll be gone in moments.

YIELD: Thirty tots

1 tablespoon onion flakes
¼ cup coconut oil, melted
½ cup arrowroot flour
¼ cup fresh herbs, chopped (basil, parsley, tarragon, chives, etc.)
¼ teaspoon unprocessed salt
Black pepper to taste
¾ cup grated raw sweet potato, tightly packed
½ cup shredded unsweetened coconut
1 tablespoon coconut oil, if frying

- In a large mixing bowl, stir together the onion flakes, coconut oil, arrowroot, herbs, salt, and pepper. Add the grated sweet potato and mix together until it forms a thick dough.
- Put ½ cup shredded coconut on a flat plate.
- Roll the dough into balls with your hands to about ½ to ¾ inches in diameter. Then roll each ball in the shredded coconut to coat the dough and make a cylinder shape. Tap lightly into the coconut on each end so the top and bottom flatten to make a cylinder shape—like a tater tot.
- To fry, melt a tablespoon of coconut oil in a large skillet over medium heat. When a drop of water flicked on the surface sizzles, it's ready. Place the dough cylinders in the hot oil and fry for 1 to 2 minutes. Watch them carefully and rotate them when the underside gets brown. Fry until all sides are golden brown, about 4 minutes. Remove finished tots to a plate covered with a paper towel.
- If you're baking them, preheat the oven to 400°F. Bake on a parchment-covered baking sheet for about 15 minutes, until golden brown. They taste delicious both ways.

VARIATION: Cauliflower Tater Tot
Follow the recipe above, substituting raw "riced" cauliflower instead of sweet potatoes. To rice the cauliflower, grate it coarsely with a box grater or process briefly in a food processor with the "S" blade.

Gluten-free	Dairy-free	Egg-free	Meat-free	Tree Nut-free	Vegan	Diabetic-friendly	Candida-friendly	High-protein	10 minutes or less
●	●	●	●	●	●	●	●		

TAMALE PIE

Here's the Mexican-style casserole, reinvented Paleo-style. It's a quick and savory breakfast with meat, spices, and a crust that tastes just like cornbread, but isn't. It's easy to prep the night before, refrigerate, and bake in the morning. You can freeze leftovers up to 3 months—just defrost overnight and bake in the morning in an oven or toaster oven. Serve with Paleo Sour Cream (page 256) and chopped cilantro.

YIELD: One 9-inch square pan; serves four • **EQUIPMENT:** A food processor is helpful but not required

FILLING:
1 tablespoon coconut oil
2 cloves garlic, diced
1 onion, diced
½ teaspoon ground cumin
½ teaspoon chili powder
⅛ teaspoon pure chipotle powder
Unprocessed salt and pepper to taste
1 pound grass-fed sausage, such as
    Spicy Chorizo (page 237) or Zesty
    Italian Sausage (page 239)
4 fresh tomatoes diced, or one small
    can pure crushed tomatoes
¼ cup cilantro, diced
1 tablespoon fresh oregano, or
    ½ teaspoon dried oregano

TAMALE DOUGH:
1 cup almond meal
¼ heaping teaspoon unprocessed salt
¼ teaspoon baking soda
2 tablespoons nutritional yeast
1⅓ cups (302 grams) Coconut Butter
    (page 33); if mixing by hand, soften butter
    by placing the container in a bowl of
    warm water
2 large eggs
2 tablespoons lemon juice
1 tablespoon onion flakes (optional)
3 tablespoons Homemade Bone Broth
    (page 47) or filtered water
¼ cup chopped cilantro to garnish

- Preheat the oven to 350°F. In a skillet heat the oil over medium-high heat. Add the garlic, onion, cumin, chili powder, chipotle powder, salt, and pepper. Sauté until the onions begin to soften, about 2 minutes.

- Add the meat and sauté until slightly browned, about 3 minutes.

- Stir in the tomatoes, cilantro, and oregano. Heat to boiling and pour the mixture into a greased 9-inch square baking pan.

continues

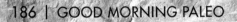

continued

- For the dough, in a mixing bowl or food processor, place the almond meal, salt, baking soda, and nutritional yeast. Add the coconut butter and mix well. Add the eggs, lemon juice, onion flakes, if using, and broth. The dough will be quite thick. If it is too thick to spread, add a bit more liquid. Spoon the dough over the filling in the pan and spread to cover the filling.

- Bake for 30 to 35 minutes, or until the dough is cooked and starting to brown. Sprinkle with chopped cilantro and serve.

Gluten-free	Dairy-free	Egg-free	Meat-free	Tree Nut–free	Vegan	Diabetic-friendly	Candida-friendly	High-protein	10 minutes or less
●	●					●	●	●	

EGG FOO YONG

My first teenage infatuation was a young Chinese art student, family friend, and frequent guest chef in our home. Fong Yiu Lee painted portraits and taught us to make authentic Cantonese dishes. Egg Foo Yong is a 5-minute breakfast, and the meat is optional. This Paleo-adapted version is a great use for leftover bits of veggies, and it tastes great without the sticky-sweet sauce. I haven't seen our friend Fong Yiu Lee since he left to paint portraits in the New Orleans French Quarter. "Egg foo yong" means "hibiscus flower eggs," referring to the delicate texture and color of this dish.

YIELD: Makes four "pancakes"; serves two

4 large eggs
1 cup vegetables, raw or cooked, such as sprouts,
    green onion, celery, bell pepper, mushrooms, parsley, kale,
    broccoli, onion, cabbage, or carrot, finely diced or shredded
1 clove garlic, chopped
Unprocessed salt and pepper to taste
½ cup chopped cooked meat, such as chicken, shrimp, or beef (optional)
2 tablespoons coconut aminos, plus more to drizzle on top
2 tablespoons coconut oil for frying
½ teaspoon toasted sesame oil to drizzle on top

- Crack the eggs into a bowl and beat with a fork or whisk. Add the vegetables, garlic, salt, pepper, optional meat, and coconut aminos. Stir briefly to combine.

- Heat the coconut oil in a nonstick skillet or wok on high heat. When the oil is fully heated, ladle one fourth of the egg mixture into the pan so that it is about 4 to 6 inches wide and thicker in the center of the pan. Let it cook for 2 to 3 minutes, then flip with a spatula and cook until golden brown and nicely puffed up. Repeat with the remaining egg mixture.

- Drizzle with coconut aminos and a bit of toasted sesame oil. Serve immediately.

Gluten-free	Dairy-free	Egg-free	Meat-free	Tree Nut-free	Vegan	Diabetic-friendly	Candida-friendly	High-protein	10 minutes or less
●	●		●	●		●	●	●	●

CAULIFLOWER FRIED RICE

You won't find this luscious dish in Chinatown. Cauliflower rice is very easy to prepare, super-low in carbs, and economical too. It makes a nourishing and satisfying breakfast. It's also a delicious vegetarian meal, as meat is optional. Freeze leftovers up to 6 weeks in BPA-free serving-size containers.

YIELD: Serves two • **EQUIPMENT:** A food processor is helpful but not required

3 tablespoons coconut or olive oil
2 cloves garlic, chopped
1-inch piece of fresh ginger root, peeled and diced
½ onion, chopped
1 carrot, cut into strips and diced, with the peel
4 ounces diced pork, ham, chicken, or turkey, in ½-inch pieces (optional)
2 whole green onions, thinly sliced on the bias
3 tablespoons liquid coconut aminos
2 large eggs, beaten
Unprocessed salt and pepper to taste
½ head cauliflower, riced (see Tip)
A handful of your favorite sprouts (optional)
1 teaspoon toasted sesame oil
1 tablespoon chopped green onion for garnish

- In a thick-bottomed skillet over high heat, place 1 tablespoon of the coconut oil. Add the garlic and ginger and cook briefly, for about 1 minute. Add the onions and cook until they begin to soften, about 2 minutes. Add the carrots and meat, if using, and cook briefly, about 2 minutes. Add the green onions and liquid aminos. Cover the pan and cook for about 1 minute until the veggies are fragrant and still a bit crisp. Transfer the mixture to a bowl and set aside.

- Cook the eggs: Return the pan to the heat. Scramble the eggs in 1 tablespoon coconut oil with salt and pepper. When they're still moist, remove them from the heat to a bowl. Break them up with a spatula and set aside.

continues

- Heat the final tablespoon of coconut oil in the pan. Add the riced cauliflower, stirring so it doesn't stick to the bottom. You may also add 1 to 2 tablespoons filtered water and cover the pan to steam the "rice" until it's al dente, as you like it, somewhere between crunchy and mushy. This will take 1 to 2 minutes.

- Assemble and serve: Add everything to the cauliflower in the pan. Veggies, eggs, meat, and sprouts, if using. Season with liquid aminos and heat everything through before serving, about 1 minute. Remove from the heat. Stir in the toasted sesame oil. Garnish with green onion and serve.

Tip: To rice cauliflower, put chunks of cauliflower into the bowl of your food processor or blender and pulse until the cauliflower is in small, rice-size pieces. Or you can grate it fine with a box grater.

Gluten-free	Dairy-free	Egg-free	Meat-free	Tree Nut-free	Vegan	Diabetic-friendly	Candida-friendly	High-protein	10 minutes or less
●	●		●	●		●	●		●

EGG DROP SOUP

While authentic egg drop soup may seem odd for breakfast, it is a tasty and a satisfying meal that you can have ready in 10 minutes flat. You can make it your own by using other veggies such as bok choy, chopped chard, or seaweed, vegetarian or with meat. The quality of this soup depends on your broth; I prefer Homemade Bone Broth (page 47), but conventional works, too.

YIELD: Serves four

1¼ cups shiitake mushrooms, thinly sliced
1 tablespoon coconut oil
4 cups Homemade Bone Broth (page 47), or use your favorite broth
½ cup cooked chicken, ham, shrimp, or beef, in ½-inch pieces (optional)
½ cup carrot, diced, with the peel
1 teaspoon peeled, grated ginger root
Unprocessed salt and pepper to taste
1 tablespoon hiziki or wakame seaweed, soaked 5 minutes in ¼ cup hot water
1 tablespoon arrowroot flour, stirred into ¼ cup cold filtered water or broth
2 teaspoons toasted sesame oil
3 large eggs, lightly beaten
3 green onions, diced

- In a medium saucepan, sauté the mushrooms in oil for about 1 minute until soft.

- Add the broth, meat (if using), carrot, ginger, salt, pepper, and seaweed. Bring to a boil, cover, and simmer for 3 minutes. Stir in the arrowroot mixture to thicken.

- Remove the pan from the heat. Add the sesame oil and eggs, stirring once briefly. The eggs will cook immediately on contact with the hot broth. Serve with chopped green onions.

Gluten-free	Dairy-free	Egg-free	Meat-free	Tree Nut-free	Vegan	Diabetic-friendly	Candida-friendly	High-protein	10 minutes or less
●	●		●	●		●	●	●	●

PHO GA, VIETNAMESE CHICKEN SOUP

Pho Ga, or chicken soup, is a favorite Vietnamese breakfast served everywhere from hotels to homes and from street carts. The quality of the broth determines the flavor and nutrients in the soup. Traditionally made with rice noodles, this recipe uses zoodles (zucchini noodles). They're quick to make with a spiral vegetable slicer, mandoline, or julienne peeler—see page 26. Make the broth ahead and freeze in flat BPA-free containers, so it's quick to defrost as you cook this easy soup.

YIELD: Serves two

3 cups Homemade Bone Broth (page 47), or use your favorite broth

1-inch piece of fresh ginger root, peeled and sliced very thin

1 clove garlic, crushed

⅛ teaspoon ground cardamom

8 ounces chicken breast, diced

1 tablespoon liquid coconut aminos (optional)

1 stick cinnamon (optional)

1 whole star anise (optional)

1 medium zucchini, sliced into thin zoodles

1 green onion, chopped

Unprocessed salt to taste, if necessary (probably not needed if aminos and broth are salted)

Black pepper to taste

OPTIONAL GARNISHES:
Fresh bean sprouts
Basil leaves
Fresh cilantro leaves
Lime wedges

- In a medium saucepan heat the broth, ginger, garlic, cardamom, chicken breast, coconut aminos, and cinnamon and anise, if using. Bring to a boil and turn the heat down to a low simmer. Cover the pan to allow the chicken to cook for 2 to 3 minutes.

- Add the zoodles, green onion, salt, and pepper to taste. Cover and simmer for 1 minute. The idea is to cook the zoodles until barely soft, but not mushy.

- Pour into two bowls and serve with optional garnishes.

Gluten-free	Dairy-free	Egg-free	Meat-free	Tree Nut-free	Vegan	Diabetic-friendly	Candida-friendly	High-protein	10 minutes or less
●	●	●		●		●	●	●	●

ZOODLE SOUP

Classic Chinese noodles with a Paleo twist, this dish is loaded with protein to keep your metabolism on track all morning. Zoodles are zucchini noodles—easily made with a spiral vegetable slicer, mandoline, or julienne peeler—see Tools (page 26). I call this "Refrigerator Noodle Soup" because it's flexible and a great way to use vegetables in the fridge. While you can use packaged broth, I find that Homemade Bone Broth (page 47) adds extra richness to the soup. I suggest keeping the broth on hand in the freezer for quick meals.

YIELD: Serves two

2 cups Homemade Bone Broth (page 47), or use your favorite broth
1 zucchini, in thin strips (zoodles)
1 carrot, in thin strips (optional)
A large handful of greens, such as kale, spinach, chard, or bok choy,
    cut in bite-size pieces
2 green onions, chopped
6 ounces any meat, such as chicken, pork, beef, natural prosciutto,
    or ham, in small pieces (optional)
1-inch piece ginger root, peeled and sliced thin
1 clove garlic, diced (optional)
Unprocessed salt and pepper to taste
1 tablespoon toasted sesame oil (optional)

- Bring the broth to a slow boil in a medium saucepan, thawing it if necessary.

- Add the zucchini and carrot strips, greens, green onion, meat (if using), ginger, garlic (if using), salt, and pepper. Bring to a boil, cover, and turn down the heat to a low simmer. Cook until the veggies are barely softened, for 2 to 4 minutes.

- Remove from the heat. Add sesame oil, if using, and serve.

Gluten-free	Dairy-free	Egg-free	Meat-free	Tree Nut–free	Vegan	Diabetic-friendly	Candida-friendly	High-protein	10 minutes or less
●	●	●	●	●	●	●	●	●	●

9

THE EGG ALWAYS COMES FIRST

*"Nobody can go back and start a new beginning,
but anyone can start today and make a new ending."*
—Anonymous

As a chef, I can confidently say that eggs are a miraculous food. A simple egg can be scrambled, fried, boiled, poached, baked, and even eaten raw—which is most likely the way our Paleolithic ancestors ate them. Just whip an egg and you'll have crepes, popovers, or a delicate soufflé. Mix eggs with coconut butter, and presto! You've got Fluffy White Bread (page 55). Make a frittata, an omelet, or Huevos Rancheros (page 209). Eggs are quick to prepare, and they make satisfying, easy breakfasts, like Cowboy Baked Eggs (page 203) or Eggs Benedict (page 208).

Eggs are a rich source of nutrients. A single egg contains 6 grams of high-quality protein and all of the nine essential amino acids. One egg yolk can provide up to 25 IU of vitamin D, a deficiency that's pandemic in the modern world. Yolks are one of the richest sources of the B-complex vitamin choline, for healthy nerve function and reduced inflammation. The high sulfur content in eggs promotes healthy hair and nails.

Many doctors suggest we go easy on eggs and avoid overindulging. Eating any food too much or too often can cause the body to build resistance, which can lead to intolerances or allergies. It's good to remember that in the ancestral diet, eggs were a seasonal food eaten only in the spring.

Healthy eggs have a thick shell that's hard to break, bright orange yolks, and a delicious flavor. But which eggs are best? It's amazing to read the enticing terms on egg cartons. Many of these terms are legally regulated. What do the labels mean?

If you don't have time to figure them out, here's a quick guide:

Pastured Organic: These are the best eggs. Pastured eggs have been shown to contain up to nineteen times more omega-3 fatty acids than supermarket eggs. Pasture-raised organic eggs are more expensive, as organic feed is GMO-free and costs more, and more space is required to raise the chickens. Find the best eggs locally from an organic farm or a farmers' market. It's great to meet your producers face-to-face. Even better is to visit the farm, meet the chickens, and gather a few eggs yourself.

Pastured: These hens must get at least 30 percent of their dry-feed from pasture grazing outside. However the other 70 percent of their diet is not regulated, and may be GMO grains.

Organic: These hens are fed a certified organic diet. This is the only category that allows no pesticides or GMO grains. Hens are uncaged; however, there is no regulation on chickens per square foot, so they may not have room to walk around. And they are not required to have outdoor access.

Free Range: Hens must be allowed some access to the outdoors. But there are no requirements as to how much time they spend outdoors, or the quality or size of the outdoor area. This term is quite vague and doesn't necessarily indicate a healthy environment or the level of crowding in the coop. "Free range" tells you nothing about the chicken's diet.

Certified Humane: Hens are uncaged and indoors, with less crowded conditions than other categories. But it doesn't indicate the hen's ability to move around, or guarantee a healthy diet.

Cage-Free: Hens live uncaged, typically indoors, and may never see daylight. Since diet is not addressed in this term, they are most likely eating GMO grains.

Vegetarian Fed: This is not a regulated term, so your guess is as good as mine.

Omega-3 Eggs: Does not necessarily indicate healthy eggs. Hens may be fed low-quality omega-3 fats that are already oxidized, which offer no health benefit or could be detrimental. Many doctors suggest you skip this and save money.

Fresh: This is not a legal term in the United States. Eggs are typically 3 weeks old by the time we find them on the grocery shelf. You'll find the freshest eggs at a local farm or from a friend with chickens. Better yet, raise your own.

Natural or Naturally Raised: This term is not regulated for chickens, so it means nothing.

ASPARAGUS FRITTATA WITH HERBS AND CREAM CHEESE

One of the first vegetables that signal the start of spring is fresh asparagus at local farmers' markets. This easy frittata makes a flavorful breakfast or brunch. Frittatas can be served hot, at room temperature, or cold. You can make them a day or an hour before and cover. So frittatas make an easy special-occasion breakfast for families or guests. Freeze leftovers up to 3 months in serving-size portions in a BPA-free container. Defrost overnight and reheat in the oven for about 30 minutes.

YIELD: Serves six

¾ pound asparagus, trimmed and cut into ½-inch chunks
10 large eggs
2 tablespoons unsweetened coconut milk (page 35) or almond milk (page 36)
Unprocessed salt and black pepper to taste
¼ cup chopped fresh herbs (green onion, parsley, tarragon, etc.)
2 tablespoons coconut oil or olive oil
¼ cup Paleo Cream Cheese (page 43), or grass-fed goat cheese, in small pieces

- To steam the asparagus, pour filtered water into a shallow pan about ¼ inch deep. Add the asparagus and bring to a boil. Turn the heat down very low, cover, and cook for about 4 minutes or until barely al dente. To stop the cooking, drain the contents into a strainer over the sink. Run cold water over it and set aside.

- In a medium mixing bowl, beat the eggs, milk, salt, pepper, and herbs. Stir in the asparagus.

- Preheat the broiler to 500°F. In a heavy ovenproof, nonstick pan, heat the oil over medium heat. Flick a few drops of water into the pan—when it sizzles, it is ready. Pour in the egg mixture and tilt the pan around to distribute the eggs evenly in the pan. As it starts cooking, lift the edge and bottom of the frittata with a spatula to allow liquid eggs to run underneath. Turn the heat down very low, cover, and cook for 8 to 10 minutes.

- Sprinkle crumbled cheese on top, and place the frittata in the broiler for 1 to 3 minutes. Watch it carefully. When the top of the eggs is barely firm, remove it from the oven. Cool in the pan for 2 minutes, then carefully slide it onto a serving platter.

Gluten-free	Dairy-free	Egg-free	Meat-free	Tree Nut–free	Vegan	Diabetic-friendly	Candida-friendly	High-protein	10 minutes or less
●	●		●	●		●	●	●	

BACON-WRAPPED EGGS

You can't eat just one of these tasty morsels! During baking, the bacon strip creates a crust around the egg and makes a tantalizing treat. They're easy to make and loaded with protein. Of course, the key ingredient is quality bacon, so opt for non-GMO bacon without preservatives or sugar if you can. These are even yummier with Cilantro Pesto (page 253) or Spicy Cheese Sauce (page 258), which you may choose to keep on hand in the freezer for a quick topping.

YIELD: Four bacon-wrapped eggs; serves two

4 slices bacon
Coconut oil and coconut flour for greasing and dusting pans
4 large eggs
1 tablespoon chopped fresh herbs, such as parsley,
    cilantro, green onion, or tarragon
2 tablespoons Spicy Cheese Sauce (page 258) (optional)

- Preheat the oven to 375°F. On a parchment-covered baking sheet, lay out the bacon strips lengthwise. Bake for about 10 minutes, or until they are almost cooked, still flexible, not crispy.

- Grease four ramekins or 4 cups of a muffin-tin and dust with coconut flour. If using a muffin tin, fill the remaining empty cups with ¼ inch of water, to prevent burning.

- Take a slice of half-cooked bacon at a time, and wrap the inside of each muffin cup to create a ring. Carefully crack an egg into the center of each bacon-lined cup. Top with chopped herbs.

- Bake for 10 to 15 minutes, until the egg whites are set. Your baking time will depend on how you like the yolks, runny or hard (see Tip).

- Remove from the oven and allow to set for 2 minutes. Place the bacon egg cups on a plate. Serve with Spicy Cheese Sauce.

Tip: If you like your yolks hard, use a sharp knife to prick the raw yolks in the muffin tins before baking.

Gluten-free	Dairy-free	Egg-free	Meat-free	Tree Nut–free	Vegan	Diabetic-friendly	Candida-friendly	High-protein	10 minutes or less
●	●			●		●		●	

CLASSIC OMELET WITH EIGHTEEN VARIATIONS

If you can scramble an egg, you can make an omelet. It's a super-quick breakfast, and there are a thousand variations. I've listed a few of my favorites to get you started. The most basic omelet is for one person, folded over, with something wonderful inside. You can repeat the process if you're serving two or more people. Use two or three eggs per person, depending on hunger level. Serve with toasted bread, Paleo Butter (page 45), and a side of Fermented Veggies (page 48). Especially yummy accompaniments are Sour Cream Onion Dill Bread (page 65) and Old-World Seed Bread (page 59).

YIELD: One omelet; serves one • **EQUIPMENT:** An 8-inch nonstick pan

2 to 3 large eggs
2 tablespoons unsweetened coconut milk (page 35) or
 almond milk (page 36)
Unprocessed salt and black pepper to taste
2 tablespoons coconut oil

- Prepare your filling and set aside. See suggestions on the next page.

- Crack the eggs into a bowl. Add milk, salt, and pepper. Beat well with a whisk or a fork until smooth.

- Heat the oil in a pan over medium-low heat. When a drop of water sizzles when flicked on the surface, it's ready. Pour in the eggs.

- Turn down the heat and cover. Do not stir. Just let the eggs cook for about 1 minute until the bottom starts to set.

- With a heat-resistant rubber spatula, gently lift one side of the egg without breaking it and allow the liquid egg to flow underneath into the bottom of the pan. Cook until it is just golden brown on the bottom and barely cooked on the top, about 2 minutes.

- Now's the time to add your filling. Spoon it in so it covers the bottom half of the circle of eggs. Gently slide the omelet onto a plate, filled side first, folding the other half over it as you go. Enjoy.

continues

OMELET FILLINGS:

Ham and Cheese—¼ cup diced natural ham, 2 tablespoons Spicy Cheese Sauce (page 258)

Bacon Avocado—Two strips cooked bacon, in small pieces, ½ avocado, sliced

Baby Spinach—1 cup raw baby spinach, wilted in garlic and olive oil

Mushrooms and Watercress—½ cup fresh sliced mushrooms, sautéed in garlic and olive oil, a handful of fresh watercress, slightly wilted

Stir-Fried Veggie—Sautéed diced veggies: ½ onion, ½ carrot, a handful of kale, a handful of mushrooms

Leftovers—A favorite! Heat up your leftovers. Spike them with Spicy Cheese Sauce (page 258).

Wild Salmon and Cream Cheese—Sauté one diced green onion with 3 ounces wild salmon. Serve with 2 tablespoons Paleo Cream Cheese (page 43) or grass-fed goat cheese.

Garden—Sauté chopped scallions, a handful of snow peas, ½ red pepper, and a handful of sunflower sprouts

Wild Mushrooms and Asparagus—Sauté ½ cup raw mushrooms in garlic and coconut oil. Add four spears asparagus and steam until tender. Garnish with parsley.

Tex-Mex—Sauté ½ sliced red onion and ¼ cup chopped tomatoes with ¼ teaspoon chili powder. Add ½ sliced avocado and 2 tablespoons Spicy Cheese Sauce (page 258).

Mediterranean—Sauté ½ onion, a handful of sliced cherry tomatoes, ½ sliced bell pepper, a handful of chopped basil, and two slices of natural prosciutto

continues

Tri-Colored—Sauté ½ cup broccoli florets, three slices of tomato, ½ onion, ½ yellow bell pepper, diced. Serve with 2 tablespoons Avocado Pesto (page 252).

Italian—Gently wilt 1 cup of raw baby spinach in garlic and coconut oil. Stir in 2 tablespoons sun-dried tomatoes. Serve with Parmesan Cheese Sauce (page 257).

Spicy Mexican—Sauté ½ onion, 1 clove garlic, 2 ounces Spicy Chorizo (page 237), 2 tablespoons tomatillos (or chopped tomatoes), with ¼ teaspoon chili powder. Serve with ½ sliced avocado, hot sauce, and Cilantro Pesto (page 253).

Asian—Sauté ½ cup sliced shiitake mushrooms with 1 clove crushed garlic and 1 teaspoon diced ginger root, 3 tablespoons sliced water chestnuts, and one diced green onion. After cooking, garnish with 1 teaspoon toasted sesame oil.

Herb with Cream Cheese—Stir into the eggs ¼ cup finely chopped fresh herbs, such as green onions or chives, parsley, basil, cilantro, tarragon, or dill. Before folding, add in 2 tablespoons crumbled Paleo Cream Cheese (page 43).

So Cal—½ cup coarsely chopped baby spinach, wilted with 1 tablespoon diced fresh basil and one chopped green onion. Garnish with sliced avocado.

Turkey Gobbler—¼ cup diced turkey meat, 2 tablespoons Homemade Bacon Bits (page 42), 2 tablespoons chopped green onion. Serve with Paleo Sour Cream (page 256).

Gluten-free	Dairy-free	Egg-free	Meat-free	Tree Nut-free	Vegan	Diabetic-friendly	Candida-friendly	High-protein	10 minutes or less
●	●			●		●	●	●	●

BAKED EGGS IN PORTOBELLO MUSHROOM WITH BACON

This appetizing breakfast is really easy to make. Portobello mushrooms are just a giant version of button mushrooms, so they're great to stuff with almost anything. Button mushrooms have grown wild since prehistoric times and were eaten by early hunter-gatherers. Romans revered mushrooms as *cibus diorum*, or "food for the gods." This recipe combines the rich, hearty flavors of portobello mushrooms, herbs, and bacon. Choose non-GMO, sugar-free bacon or prosciutto if possible. For a tasty side dish, try Fermented Veggies (page 48).

YIELD: Serves two

2 portobello mushrooms
2 tablespoons coconut or olive oil
Unprocessed salt and black pepper to taste
⅓ cup chopped green onions
3 tablespoons Homemade Bacon Bits (page 42),
    cooked bacon pieces, or two slices natural prosciutto
2 large eggs

- Preheat the oven to 375°F. Cover a baking sheet with parchment paper.

- Rinse and pat dry the mushrooms, removing any dirt. Break or cut the stem off at its base. Brush the mushrooms with olive oil and sprinkle with salt and pepper. Place them on the baking sheet cap side down, with the gill side facing up. It's important that they don't tip over. You may trim the cap side of the mushroom so it stays level and will hold the egg without spilling.

- Sprinkle half of the green onions over the mushrooms and add the bacon bits.

- Make a well in the center of the herbs and meat, and carefully crack an egg into each mushroom. Prick the raw yolks if you like your yolks hard.

- Bake for 25 to 35 minutes, according to how you like your eggs.

- Allow to cool for 5 minutes. Sprinkle with the remaining green onions and season with salt and pepper as needed. Enjoy!

Gluten-free	Dairy-free	Egg-free	Meat-free	Tree Nut-free	Vegan	Diabetic-friendly	Candida-friendly	High-protein	10 minutes or less
●	●			●		●		●	

COWBOY BAKED EGGS

This is a casserole with spinach, bacon, and avocado that you might cook outside on a campfire. It's a powerhouse of phytonutrients, protein, and honest flavor. Assemble it in just a few minutes and pop in the oven as you get ready to start your day. Three cups of spinach sounds like a lot, however it bakes down into a soft bed of greens. Look for bacon that's non-GMO and sugar-free if possible. You can also assemble this in the evening, refrigerate, and bake in the morning. Cut it into squares and freeze leftovers individually wrapped for future cowboy meals. Try it with Bacon Chili Cornbread muffins (page 71) and Paleo Sour Cream (page 256). Also try it with a side of Fermented Veggies (page 48).

YIELD: One 9-inch square pan; serves four

8 ounces raw bacon, cut in ½-inch pieces
8 ounces fresh baby spinach, about 3 cups
6 large eggs
2 tablespoons coconut milk (page 35) or filtered water
¼ teaspoon chili powder
Unprocessed salt and pepper to taste
1 avocado, pitted, peeled, and sliced
6 cherry tomatoes, halved

- Preheat the oven to 350°F. Grease a 9-inch square baking pan.

- In a large skillet over medium heat, cook the bacon for 3 to 4 minutes, stirring occasionally, until crispy.

- Put all the baby spinach into the baking dish.

- Pour the bacon and bacon fat over the spinach and stir it in a bit.

- Whisk the eggs in a bowl, adding the coconut milk, chili powder, and salt and pepper to taste. Slowly pour the eggs over the spinach in the baking pan. Gently stir the spinach around a bit to mix the eggs in.

- Just before baking, top with avocado slices and cherry tomatoes in rows.

- Bake for 18 to 22 minutes, or until eggs are firm.

- Cut into squares and serve.

Gluten-free	Dairy-free	Egg-free	Meat-free	Tree Nut-free	Vegan	Diabetic-friendly	Candida-friendly	High-protein	10 minutes or less
●	●			●		●		●	

ITALIAN BAKED EGGS

This luscious Italian breakfast is easy to make and beautiful to serve—see photo in the insert. It's a colorful layering of onions, zucchini, and eggs with rich Parmesan Cheese Sauce (page 257) that's completely dairy-free. It is called *Uova al forno con pomodoro e zucchini*, or "Baked eggs in the oven with tomato and zucchini." These eggs are wonderful plain or with Garlic Naan (page 78). Buon appetito!

YIELD: Serves two

2 tablespoons olive oil
2 cloves garlic, minced
½ onion cut in thin half-moons
1 large zucchini, or 2 small ones, sliced thin
Unprocessed salt and black pepper to taste
1 ripe Roma tomato, sliced thin
1 tablespoon chopped fresh basil, or 1 teaspoon dried basil
4 large eggs
1 recipe Parmesan Cheese Sauce (page 257)
Basil to garnish

- Preheat the oven to 350°F. In an ovenproof nonstick skillet over medium heat, heat the olive oil. Add the garlic and onions. Sauté briefly until they begin to soften, about 2 minutes.

- Add the zucchini, salt, and pepper. Sauté briefly until the zucchini begins to soften and most of the liquids cook away, about 2 to 4 minutes.

- Remove the pan from the heat. Arrange the tomato slices and basil sprinkles on top of the zucchini. Make four wells with your fingers, and break the eggs into the wells.

- Place the pan in the oven and bake for 15 to 20 minutes, until the egg whites are just barely cooked.

- Meanwhile, in a small blender, prepare the Parmesan Cheese sauce.

- When the eggs are cooked, remove the pan from the oven. Pour the Parmesan Cheese Sauce over everything. Garnish with chopped basil and serve.

Gluten-free	Dairy-free	Egg-free	Meat-free	Tree Nut–free	Vegan	Diabetic-friendly	Candida-friendly	High-protein	10 minutes or less
●	●		●	●		●	●	●	

MEDITERRANEAN EGGS WITH SPINACH AND SAUSAGE

This high-protein, low-carb, one-skillet meal has a real Roman or Sicilian flavor when you use Zesty Italian Sausage (page 239). Fresh herbs add exquisite flavor if you have them; or substitute half the amount of dry herbs. Homemade Spicy Cheese Sauce (page 258) adds a rich flavor that's completely dairy-free.

YIELD: Serves two

2 tablespoons olive oil
2 cloves garlic, minced
½ onion, diced
2 patties Zesty Italian Sausage (page 239), or your favorite Italian sausage
1 teaspoon fresh rosemary (optional)
1 tablespoon chopped fresh tarragon (optional)
2 tablespoons chopped fresh parsley (optional)
Unprocessed salt to taste
Black pepper to taste
2 to 3 cups raw baby spinach, coarsely chopped
⅓ cup Spicy Cheese Sauce (page 258) (optional)
2 Roma tomatoes, diced
4 large eggs
1 tablespoon chopped parsley for garnish

- Preheat the oven to 375°F. In an ovenproof skillet over medium heat, heat the olive oil. Add the garlic, onion, sausage, and herbs, if using. Sauté briefly until they begin to soften, about 2 minutes. Add salt and pepper to taste, depending on the flavor in your sausage.

- Remove the pan from the heat. Put the spinach into the pan over the sausage—it will be very high, but don't worry, it will cook down a lot. Spoon the Spicy Cheese Sauce on top of the spinach, if using. Then add the diced tomatoes. Make four egg-size holes with a spoon, and break the eggs into the holes. Bake for 15 to 20 minutes, just until the egg whites are cooked, but not overdone. Garnish with chopped parsley and serve.

Gluten-free	Dairy-free	Egg-free	Meat-free	Tree Nut-free	Vegan	Diabetic-friendly	Candida-friendly	High-protein	10 minutes or less
●	●			●		●	●	●	

GREEK EGG "EYES"

If you live in Athens or the Greek Islands, you'll find this easy everyday breakfast on the street corners. The recipe is from my friend Kalpita in Athens, who says it will stave off a big fat Greek hunger all morning. The name Αυγά μάτια means "egg eyes," like two eggs looking up at you, served with a side salad of Kalamata olives and tomatoes. Oregano adds a high-nutrition punch to this breakfast, as it is packed with antioxidants, vitamin K, iron, manganese, and antibacterial benefits. Paleo Feta Cheese (page 44) is a yummy addition—you can make it ahead and keep it on hand in the freezer for lots of other uses. Or substitute grass-fed goat cheese.

YIELD: Serves one

1 small tomato, sliced
½ cucumber, sliced
2 tablespoons Kalamata olives, coarsely chopped
3 tablespoons Paleo Feta Cheese (page 44), or grass-fed goat cheese, crumbled
2 teaspoons fresh oregano, diced, or ½ teaspoon dried oregano
2 to 3 tablespoons extra-virgin, first-pressed olive oil
2 large eggs
Unprocessed salt and pepper to taste

- On the side of a large plate, toss together the tomato, cucumber, olives, feta cheese, and oregano. Drizzle them with 1 tablespoon of the olive oil.

- Heat 1 to 2 tablespoons olive oil in a small nonstick pan over medium heat. When a drop of water flicked into the pan sizzles, it's ready. To fry the eggs, break two eggs into the pan so that they retain a nice rounded shape and do not spread out too much. Add salt and pepper. Fry for a couple of minutes or until the whites are firm. Many Greeks like their yolks cooked through, so they spoon a bit of hot olive oil from the side of the pan over the yolks several times. When the eggs are as you like them, slide them onto the plate next to the vegetables, like two eyes looking up at you.

Gluten-free	Dairy-free	Egg-free	Meat-free	Tree Nut-free	Vegan	Diabetic-friendly	Candida-friendly	High-protein	10 minutes or less
●	●		●	●		●	●	●	●

EGG SANDWICH MADE EASY

Sometimes, the best way to start off the day is with a breakfast sandwich. Based on an American fast-food classic, this is the perfect combination of Paleo muffin, eggs, sausage, and cheese on-the-go. I love the convenience of grabbing a finished breakfast from my freezer and baking it. Or, take it with you and have breakfast at work. See make-ahead tips below to prepare several sandwiches at a time and freeze.

YIELD: Serves one

1 English muffin (page 67)
1 large egg
1 pat of Paleo Butter (page 45)
1 slice natural ham or prosciutto, or 2 slices bacon, or 1 patty
   Homemade Breakfast Sausage (page 235) (optional)
1 tablespoon Spicy Cheese Sauce (page 258) (optional)

- Toast the English muffin.

- Cook the egg as you like it—over easy, baked, scrambled, or poached.

- To assemble the sandwich, spread a bit of Paleo butter on the English muffin. Add the egg, meat, and Spicy Cheese Sauce, if using. Wrap in a paper towel and head for the door. You're off to a great start with a delicious breakfast in hand.

Make-ahead tips:
You can bake six to twelve eggs at a time in a well-greased muffin tin, jumbo muffin tin, or ramekins. Break the yolks before cooking so they cook evenly all through without a mess. Add salt and pepper. Bake for 15 to 25 minutes.

Wrap all the sandwiches tightly in wax paper and put in resealable bags for freezing. Defrost in the refrigerator overnight, and heat in the oven for 15 to 20 minutes before breakfast.

Gluten-free	Dairy-free	Egg-free	Meat-free	Tree Nut–free	Vegan	Diabetic-friendly	Candida-friendly	High-protein	10 minutes or less
●	●			●		●	●	●	●

EGGS BENEDICT

Don't be intimidated by this recipe for classic Eggs Benny. It's super-quick with blender hollandaise and easy English Muffins (page 67), so any Paleo beginner can enjoy the sumptuous flavors. See photo in the insert and check out the yummy variations below!

YIELD: Serves four • **EQUIPMENT:** Any blender (to make Hollandaise Sauce and Paleo Butter)

4 large eggs
2 English Muffins (page 67), or 4 slices Fluffy White Bread (page 55)
2 ounces Paleo Butter (page 45), or grass-fed butter
4 handfuls of baby arugula
4 slices natural prosciutto
1 recipe Hollandaise Sauce (page 254)
1 tablespoon diced herbs: chives, green onion, parsley, or tarragon

- To poach the eggs, put 1 inch of filtered water in a shallow pan and bring to a boil. One at a time, crack each egg into a separate small bowl and then slip it into the hot water. (You can also place English muffin rings into the water, and crack the eggs gently into them to hold a round shape.) As the water resumes simmering, add the second egg. Repeat for the third and fourth eggs. Remove the pan from the heat, cover, and let it sit undisturbed for 4 minutes. A poached egg is done when the whites are solid, and the yolk is still soft in the center (unless you like them hard-cooked through). As they finish, remove each egg with a slotted spoon onto a towel.

- To assemble, toast the English muffin halves and spread with butter. Put a handful of baby arugula on each one. Top with a slice of ham. Put a poached egg on top, and drizzle Hollandaise Sauce over everything. Garnish with herbs. Eat and enjoy!

VARIATIONS:
Instead of prosciutto or ham, use wild salmon, rib-eye steak, or chicken breast.

Instead of baby arugula, use baby spinach, Roma tomato, and avocado, sliced.

Instead of English Muffins, serve on portobello mushrooms or Pumpernickel Rye Bread (page 61).

Gluten-free	Dairy-free	Egg-free	Meat-free	Tree Nut-free	Vegan	Diabetic-friendly	Candida-friendly	High-protein	10 minutes or less
●	●			●		●	●	●	

HUEVOS RANCHEROS

Typical Huevos Rancheros, made with beans, corn, and cheese, aren't Paleo. Well, here's a healthy Paleo adaptation of that Mexican favorite, using refried sweet potatoes and grain-free tortillas. Meat is optional. Topped with egg, avocado, cilantro, and salsa, it's an even tastier and heartier dish. You can freeze leftover sweet potatoes in a BPA-free container.

YIELD: Serves six

REFRIED SWEET POTATOES:
2 tablespoons coconut or olive oil
½ onion, chopped
3 cloves garlic, chopped
1 teaspoon chili powder
⅛ teaspoon pure chipotle powder
¾ teaspoon ground cumin
½ pound sausage, such as Spicy Chorizo (page 237) or Homemade Breakfast Sausage (page 235) (optional)
8 ounces mushrooms, finely chopped
1 sweet potato, raw, peeled, and coarsely grated
2 tablespoons nutritional yeast

2 tablespoons lemon juice
¼ cup (57 grams) Coconut Butter (page 33)
Unprocessed salt and pepper to taste
¼ cup filtered water

HUEVOS:
1 recipe Easy Burrito Wraps (page 76), Plantain Tortillas (page 75), or Chia Corn Tortillas (page 73)
6 large eggs, fried
½ cup of your favorite tomato salsa
1 avocado, pitted, peeled, and sliced
1 recipe Spicy Cheese Sauce (page 258)
Large handful cilantro, chopped

- For the refried sweet potatoes, heat the oil in a large skillet over medium heat. Add the onion, garlic, chili powder, chipotle powder, and cumin. Sauté briefly, for about 2 minutes. If using, add sausage, and cook for another 5 minutes. Add the mushrooms and sauté briefly, for about 2 minutes. Add the sweet potato, nutritional yeast, lemon juice, coconut butter, salt, and pepper. Pour the water into the bottom of the pan. Cover to allow the sweet potato to steam for 2 to 3 minutes, stirring occasionally. When the sweet potato is soft but not mushy, remove from the heat.

- To assemble, place the wraps on serving plates. Spread the Refried Sweet Potatoes on the wraps. Add the fried egg on top. Top it with salsa, avocado slices, Spicy Cheese Sauce, and cilantro.

Gluten-free	Dairy-free	Egg-free	Meat-free	Tree Nut-free	Vegan	Diabetic-friendly	Candida-friendly	High-protein	10 minutes or less
●	●		●	●		●		●	

MUSHROOM CHEESE SOUFFLÉ

My dad was an inspired cook and the best soufflé maker in the family. His soufflé breakfasts were unforgettable, not only because of his amazing recipe, but also because he read his favorite poetry aloud to us while we ate. This recipe is a dairy-free, Paleo adaptation of my Dad's famous soufflé. I think it's every bit as delicious because, with just one bite, I hear his voice reading. Try these with Sour Cream Onion Dill Bread (page 65) and Paleo Butter (page 45).

YIELD: Two 12-ounce soufflés; serves two • **EQUIPMENT:** An electric mixer or a strong arm and a whisk

Coconut oil and coconut flour for greasing ramekins
1 tablespoon coconut oil
1 small clove garlic, chopped
2 ounces shiitake mushrooms, sliced
4 large eggs, separated

3 tablespoons full-fat unsweetened coconut milk (page 13)
1 tablespoon lemon juice
1 tablespoon nutritional yeast
⅛ teaspoon ground nutmeg
Unprocessed salt and pepper to taste

- Preheat the oven to 375°F. Grease two 12-ounce ramekins with coconut oil and dust with coconut flour.

- In a sauté pan over medium heat, place the oil. Sauté the garlic briefly, for 1 minute. Add the mushrooms, sauté until they begin to soften, about 2 minutes, and set aside.

- In a small mixing bowl, whisk together the egg yolks, coconut milk, lemon juice, nutritional yeast, nutmeg, salt, and pepper. Mix well until smooth. Stir in the mushrooms.

- Beat the egg whites in a large mixing bowl with an electric mixer or a whisk. Beat to stiff peaks, but not dry.

- Pour the egg yolk mixture into the beaten egg whites. Gently fold them together with a spatula. Pour into the baking dishes.

- Bake until tall and golden brown on top, 24 to 28 minutes. Do not open the oven door to peek, as they may fall. Serve immediately, as soufflés are most delicious hot, and generally fall within a few minutes.

Gluten-free	Dairy-free	Egg-free	Meat-free	Tree Nut–free	Vegan	Diabetic-friendly	Candida-friendly	High-protein	10 minutes or less
●	●		●	●		●	●	●	

PORTOBELLO SCRAMBLE

Portobello mushrooms have an especially rich and deep flavor. The mature version of everyday button mushrooms, they're called "Champignon de Paris" in France. My father used to collect wild mushroom in the woods near our house and bring them home to fry with scrambled eggs for breakfast. This is a super-easy recipe that reminds me of that fresh, earthy mushroom flavor. It tastes heavenly with any toasted Paleo bread, such as Old-World Seed Bread (page 59) or Pumpernickel Rye Bread (page 61).

YIELD: Serves four

2 tablespoons coconut oil or olive oil
1 clove garlic, crushed or diced
½ onion, sliced in half-moons
Unprocessed salt and pepper to taste
1 portobello mushroom, cut in fairly large pieces, about 1-inch cubes
3 leaves fresh greens, such as spinach, kale, or chard, coarsely chopped
1 tablespoon filtered water
6 large eggs, beaten
1 tablespoon nutritional yeast
1 tomato, cut in ½-inch pieces
2 tablespoons chopped parsley

- In a large nonstick skillet over medium heat, heat the oil until a drop of water sizzles. Add the garlic, onion, salt, and pepper. Sauté for about 2 minutes until the onions begin to soften, stirring occasionally.

- Add the portobello mushroom and sauté it briefly for about 2 minutes, not too long, or it will turn to mush.

- Stir in the greens, add the water, cover the pan, and turn the heat down to low, so the greens steam-cook without burning. When the greens begin to soften, after 2 to 4 minutes, stir in the beaten eggs and sprinkle in the nutritional yeast, tomato, and parsley. Scramble the eggs as you like them—some like them runny and some like them firm. Add salt and pepper to taste. Serve!

Gluten-free	Dairy-free	Egg-free	Meat-free	Tree Nut–free	Vegan	Diabetic-friendly	Candida-friendly	High-protein	10 minutes or less
●	●		●	●		●		●	●

SCRAMBLED EGGS FLORENTINE WITH CREAM CHEESE

Eggs Florentine sounds fancy, but it's just eggs over wilted greens. Of course in Florence they poach their eggs. However I like them scrambled because it's quicker—you can do them any way you like. Coconut butter and lemon gives a rich taste of cream cheese that sends this dish over the top. Use your favorite greens. Spinach cooks quickest. Kale, collards, bok choy, etc., will work too, and you'll need to adjust the cooking time. You'll need two medium skillets, preferably nonstick—one for the eggs and the other for the greens. If you cook them at the same time, you'll have breakfast in 5 minutes! Fermented Veggies (page 48) taste terrific on the side.

YIELD: Serves two

4 large eggs
2 tablespoons unsweetened coconut milk (page 35) or almond milk (page 36), or filtered water
2 tablespoons (28 grams) Coconut Butter (page 33)
1½ tablespoons lemon juice

2 handfuls of chopped fresh herbs, such as 1 green onion, dill, or parsley
Unprocessed salt and pepper to taste
2 tablespoons coconut or olive oil
1 clove garlic, diced
3 cups fresh baby spinach or equivalent greens

- In a medium mixing bowl, whisk together the eggs, milk, coconut butter, lemon juice, herbs, salt, and pepper. Don't worry if there are lumps.

- Place a tablespoon of the coconut oil in a skillet over medium heat. Add the garlic and sauté very briefly, about 1 minute. Add the spinach, salt, and pepper. Toss it all together and cover the pan. Cook the greens very briefly to wilt, without cooking away the nutrients, about 2 to 4 minutes. Add a tablespoon or two of filtered water to the pan and cover, to steam the greens another minute or two. When they're barely wilted, turn off the flame.

- In a second skillet, place the remaining 1 tablespoon of coconut oil and heat over medium heat. When a drop of water flicked on the pan sizzles, it's ready. Add the whisked eggs. Turn the heat down and stir well with a heat-resistant spatula to scramble the eggs for 2 to 3 minutes until they are to your liking—some like them runny, some like them hard.

- Serve immediately, spinach on the bottom, scrambled eggs on top.

Gluten-free	Dairy-free	Egg-free	Meat-free	Tree Nut-free	Vegan	Diabetic-friendly	Candida-friendly	High-protein	10 minutes or less
●	●		●	●		●	●	●	●

SCRAMBLED EGGS WITH CHEESE

Here's a simple recipe for cheesy eggs you can make in 5 minutes. Just whisk the eggs with these magical Paleolithic ingredients: coconut butter, lemon juice, nutritional yeast, and presto! You've got dairy-free cheese scramble. Serve plain, with toasted Old-World Seed Bread (page 59), or on Garlic Naan (page 78), with a side of Fermented Veggies (page 48).

YIELD: Serves two hungry persons

6 large eggs
½ teaspoon unprocessed salt
2 tablespoons nutritional yeast
¼ cup (57 grams) Coconut Butter (page 33)
¼ cup unsweetened coconut milk (page 35), almond milk (page 36),
   or filtered water
1½ to 2 tablespoons lemon juice
3 tablespoons coconut or olive oil

OPTIONAL ADDITIONS:
1 green onion, diced
¼ cup Homemade Bacon Bits (page 42), or cook bacon in small pieces
½ cup leftover cooked veggies, chopped

- In a large mixing bowl, whisk together the eggs, salt, nutritional yeast, coconut butter, milk, and lemon juice. Mix well and don't worry about lumps.

- In a large nonstick skillet over medium heat, heat the coconut oil until a drop of water sizzles when flicked into the pan. Pour the eggs into the pan and turn down the heat. Add the optional ingredients. Scramble the eggs for 2 to 3 minutes until they are to your liking—some like them runny, some like them firm. Serve immediately.

Gluten-free	Dairy-free	Egg-free	Meat-free	Tree Nut-free	Vegan	Diabetic-friendly	Candida-friendly	High-protein	10 minutes or less
●	●		●	●		●	●	●	●

SOFT–BOILED EGGS WITH MUSHROOMS ON TOAST

As a child my favorite breakfast was wild mushrooms sautéed in butter on toast. This is quick to make and you can use your favorite mushrooms, such as button, crimini, shiitake, maitake, etc. Soft-boiled eggs take 6 minutes to cook, so you'll need to start them before the mushrooms. And if you have made ahead some Paleo bread, your meal is a snap. This tastes wonderful with Rosemary Olive Bread (page 63).

YIELD: Serves two

4 large eggs
2 tablespoons coconut oil
1 small clove garlic, diced (optional)
6 ounces shiitake mushrooms, sliced
A handful of chopped parsley
1 tablespoon liquid coconut aminos
1 teaspoon lemon juice (optional)
Unprocessed salt and pepper to taste
4 pieces toasted Paleo bread

- To make soft-boiled eggs, fill a small saucepan half-full with water and bring to a rolling boil. Turn heat down to medium. Using a large spoon, carefully immerse the eggs completely one at a time into the boiling water. Set the timer for 6 minutes.

- In a large skillet over medium heat, place the coconut oil. Sauté the garlic very briefly, about 1 minute, and add the mushrooms. Sauté for 2 to 3 minutes until they soften. Add the parsley, coconut aminos, lemon juice (if using), salt, and pepper. If the mushrooms seem dry, stir in a bit of filtered water, and cook for 1 to 2 minutes more. Then remove from the heat.

- To open soft-boiled eggs, immerse them in cold water to stop cooking. Use a table knife to give the shell a light whack around the equator of each egg. Then lift off the top of the egg. Serve in the half shell, or scoop it out.

- Spoon the mushrooms over the toast. If the eggs are scooped out, put them on top. Or if the eggs are still in the shell, serve them on the side for a hungry eater to scoop out.

Gluten-free	Dairy-free	Egg-free	Meat-free	Tree Nut–free	Vegan	Diabetic-friendly	Candida-friendly	High-protein	10 minutes or less
●	●		●	●		●	●	●	●

SOUTHWEST FRITTATA

I'll wake up any day for spicy baked eggs with avocado and peppers. This is a colorful, open-faced omelet that starts on the stovetop and finishes in the oven. It's a snap to make, and the meat is optional. Try it with Avocado Pesto (page 252) or Cilantro Pesto (page 253). To freeze leftovers, wrap individual servings in airtight plastic wrap in a freezer container. Defrost overnight in the refrigerator and heat for 15 minutes in the oven.

YIELD: Serves two

3 tablespoons coconut oil or olive oil
1 clove garlic, diced
½ onion sliced in half-moons
6 ounces Homemade Breakfast Sausage (page 235),
   or your favorite sausage (optional)
⅛ teaspoon chili powder, or ground cumin
1 red bell pepper, in thin slices
2 green onions, diced
4 large eggs
2 tablespoons coconut milk (page 35) or filtered water
Unprocessed salt and black pepper to taste
½ avocado, pitted, peeled, and sliced
2 tablespoons fresh chopped cilantro

- Preheat the oven to 350°F. In a large nonstick, ovenproof skillet over medium heat, place the oil. Sauté the garlic and onion briefly until they begin to soften, about 2 minutes. Add the sausage, if using, and sauté about 2 minutes, just enough to barely cook it. Stir in the chili power, sweet red pepper, and green onions and continue to cook for 2 more minutes.

- In a small mixing bowl, beat the eggs with the coconut milk, salt, and pepper. When the sweet red pepper is beginning to soften, pour the eggs on top of everything, cover, and turn down the heat. Cook for about 2 minutes on top of the stove.

- Remove the cover and place in the oven, baking for about 5 minutes, until the eggs are just barely cooked on top, not overcooked. Top with sliced avocado and chopped cilantro and serve immediately.

Gluten-free	Dairy-free	Egg-free	Meat-free	Tree Nut-free	Vegan	Diabetic-friendly	Candida-friendly	High-protein	10 minutes or less
●	●		●	●		●	●	●	

SUNNY EGGS WITH GREENS AND MUSHROOMS

This one-pan breakfast is hearty with fresh greens, eggs, and crumbled Paleo Cream Cheese (or substitute soft goat cheese). I make it for special occasions because it has a gourmet flavor, yet it's really quick to prepare. Mushrooms add a full-bodied flavor—use your favorite variety, such as button, crimini, or shiitake. Steaming greens is faster than frying and protects valuable nutrients. Use your favorite leafy greens, such as kale, collard, leek, or mixed greens. I like it with leek because the mild onion flavor blends beautifully with eggs and Paleo Cream Cheese (page 43).

YIELD: Serves four

2 tablespoons coconut oil
2 cloves fresh garlic, minced or crushed
6 ounces sliced mushrooms (optional)
Unprocessed salt and pepper to taste
6 cups fresh kale (cut into ¾-inch pieces), or collard, leek, or mixed greens
2 tablespoons filtered water, if necessary to steam
4 large eggs
¼ cup crumbled Paleo Cream Cheese (page 43), or your favorite goat cheese

- In a large skillet, heat the coconut oil over medium heat. Add the garlic and cook very briefly, about 1 minute. Add the mushrooms, salt, and pepper. Cook for 3 to 4 minutes until they begin to soften. Add the greens and cover to steam the greens, stirring occasionally. If the pan dries out, add the water to steam-cook the greens briefly, about 2 to 5 minutes, depending on the greens you use.

- Just when the greens begin to wilt but are not fully cooked, make 4 wells. Crack an egg into each well and turn the heat down to low. Add salt and pepper, cover, and cook for 2 to 3 minutes. Watch carefully and if the pan dries out, add a bit more water. Cook until the eggs are as you like them—soft (about 3 minutes), or cooked through (4 to 5 minutes). Garnish with crumbled Paleo Cream Cheese and serve.

Tip: If you premake the Paleo Cream Cheese and freeze it, it will crumble nicely. You can just spoon out a bit to sprinkle on top of your greens.

Gluten-free	Dairy-free	Egg-free	Meat-free	Tree Nut-free	Vegan	Diabetic-friendly	Candida-friendly	High-protein	10 minutes or less
●	●		●	●		●	●	●	●

QUICHES

"All happiness depends on a leisurely breakfast."
—John Gunther

Quiche is French, right? Nope. The word "quiche" comes from German "kuchen," meaning *cake*. It originated in the Alsace Lorraine region, once called Lothringen in Germany, where French and German dialects embraced each other. The original quiche was an egg custard baked in brioche dough instead of a pie crust. I chose seven of my favorite quiche recipes for this book.

Here are a few tips for a perfect quiche. You can bake your quiche in a 9-inch pie pan with a crust. Or you can skip the crust and use any recipe to make mini quiches in a 12-cup muffin tin.

Quiche is an ideal make-ahead breakfast, as it holds up well. You can even make it a day ahead. Traditionally quiches can be served cold, room temperature, or warm. Store leftover quiche in individual portions in a BPA-free storage container for up to 3 months. Oh, the convenience you'll enjoy! Just defrost overnight. Then reheat in a 300°F oven for about 20 minutes, until just warm to the touch.

There are three parts to a quiche: Crust, Filling, and the Egg Custard. For the crust, use the recipe for Perfect Coconut Pie Crust (page 46).

The filling consists of vegetables and/or meats. These need to be cooked and fairly dry, meaning they have released their moisture, otherwise your quiche could be too soggy. A good rule of thumb is to have 1 to 2 cups cooked filling, depending on how creamy or solid you prefer your quiche. Like omelets, quiches are a great way to use up leftover veggies. They taste great with just about any filling—a few favorites are ham, bacon, onions, mushrooms, zucchini, asparagus, spinach, and tomatoes.

For a Paleo custard, use dairy-free, full-fat canned coconut milk and eggs. I don't use coconut beverages in a carton, as they are too thin and often contain sweeteners or additives. For a truly nutrient-dense quiche, use my favorite High-Protein Coconut Milk (page 35). You need just enough eggs to set the milk, but not so many that the quiche becomes rubbery and stiff. It's ok to have a bit of wobble in your quiche as it comes out of the oven. It is important to have all the ingredients at room temperature, so that your filling bakes completely before the crust gets too brown. To slow down browning, you can gently open the oven after about 20 minutes of baking, and brush the edges of the crust with a bit of cold water.

Tip: If you're making mini quiches without meat, it's helpful to sprinkle a teaspoon of shredded coconut in the bottom of each cup, to create a barrier so it's easy to remove them from the tin.

MINI BROCCOLI CHEESE QUICHES

These easy vegetarian quiches are filled with broccoli, eggs, and flavorful Paleo cheese, which is simply coconut butter, lemon, and nutritional yeast. I like to use the whole broccoli—stems and all, as the stems have more nutrients than the flower. Mini quiches are easy to make ahead the night before, refrigerate, and bake in the morning. Serve them right in the ramekins, and you'll never miss the crust. See tips for a perfect quiche, page 217. For storing, remove from its ramekin, wrap in plastic wrap, and freeze for a healthy grab-and-go breakfast.

YIELD: Four mini quiches in ramekins • **EQUIPMENT:** A blender or food processor is helpful but not required

- 2 tablespoons coconut oil, to grease ramekins
- 1 bunch fresh broccoli, including the stems
- 6 large eggs at room temperature
- ½ cup unsweetened full-fat coconut milk (page 13)

- Unprocessed salt and pepper to taste
- ⅛ teaspoon ground nutmeg
- 2 tablespoons lemon juice
- 1 tablespoon nutritional yeast
- 1 tablespoon Coconut Butter (page 33); if mixing by hand, soften butter by placing the container in a bowl of warm water

- Preheat the oven to 350°F. Grease four 8-ounce ramekins with coconut oil and dust with coconut flour.

- Remove the broccoli stems, peel with a paring knife, slice lengthwise, and then crosswise into ¼-inch pieces. Cut the broccoli florets into bite-size pieces.

- Pour 1 inch of water in a large saucepan and bring to a boil. Add the broccoli, bring to a boil again, and turn the heat down to simmer for 2 minutes. Drain the water; you should have about 2 cups half-cooked broccoli.

- In a mixing bowl, blender, or food processor, whisk together the eggs, coconut milk, salt, pepper, nutmeg, lemon juice, nutritional yeast, and coconut butter.

- Place the broccoli pieces in the ramekins—about ½ cup broccoli for each one. Place the ramekins on a baking sheet that's rimmed, to avoid slipping. Pour the egg mixture into the ramekins over the broccoli, dividing evenly. Bake for 35 to 40 minutes until golden brown. Serve immediately in the ramekins.

Gluten-free	Dairy-free	Egg-free	Meat-free	Tree Nut-free	Vegan	Diabetic-friendly	Candida-friendly	High-protein	10 minutes or less
●	●		●	●		●	●		

MINI VEGGIE AND HAM QUICHES

A simple breakfast in a muffin cup is a great grab-and-go meal. Chock full of vegetables, these quiches taste like an egg muffin with cheese. Freeze them, so there's never a time when you're frantic for a healthy meal. A bit of shredded coconut on the bottom helps the muffins come out of the tins easily. You can prep the ingredients in the evening, and bake in the morning. See tips for a perfect quiche, page 217. Serve hot or room temperature.

YIELD: Twelve mini quiches

¼ cup shredded unsweetened coconut flakes
1 bunch green onions, diced
½ carrot, grated, with the peel
1 handful of chopped green herbs, such as parsley,
    cilantro, or baby arugula
6 ounces ham or prosciutto, diced (optional)
½ cup almond meal
½ teaspoon baking powder
¼ heaping teaspoon unprocessed salt
Black pepper to taste
9 large eggs
1 cup unsweetened coconut milk (page 35)
1 tablespoon nutritional yeast
1 tablespoon lemon juice

• Preheat the oven to 350°F. Grease and flour a 12-muffin tin with coconut oil and coconut flour.

• Layer into the bottom of each muffin tin: shredded coconut, green onion, carrot, and herbs. Add meat, if using. Use a spoon to push the filling away from the edges of the muffin cups. This helps the eggs fill in the sides for a pretty muffin shape.

• In a mixing bowl, blender, or food processor, place the almond meal, baking powder, salt, pepper, eggs, coconut milk, nutritional yeast, and lemon juice. Mix well. Slowly pour the batter into the muffin tins. Fill them all the way to the top.

• Bake for 24 to 28 minutes, or until lightly browned.

Gluten-free	Dairy-free	Egg-free	Meat-free	Tree Nut-free	Vegan	Diabetic-friendly	Candida-friendly	High-protein	10 minutes or less
●	●					●	●		

BACON ZUCCHINI QUICHE

Quiche with bacon and zucchini makes for a savory, high-protein breakfast. Bacon adds a wholesome flavor—look for meat that's non-GMO and sugar-free if possible. Quiche is easy to prep the night before, refrigerate, and bake in the morning. It's a make-ahead dream meal, because you can freeze individually wrapped portions for another day. Then defrost overnight and bake for 20 minutes. You can also skip the crust and bake it in greased muffin cups for mini quiches. See tips for a perfect quiche, page 217. This tastes divine with Paleo Sour Cream (page 256).

YIELD: One 9-inch quiche • **EQUIPMENT:** A blender or food processor is helpful but not required

1 recipe Perfect Coconut Pie Crust (page 46)

1 tablespoon coconut oil or bacon fat

2 small onions, chopped, about 1½ cups

2 medium zucchini sliced in quarters ⅛ inch thick (¾ pound)

½ cup Homemade Bacon Bits (page 42), or 6 slices cooked bacon, in small chunks, or prosciutto

¼ teaspoon unprocessed salt to taste

¼ teaspoon black pepper to taste

5 large eggs at room temperature

½ cup unsweetened full-fat coconut milk (page 13)

½ teaspoon ground mustard

2 tablespoons nutritional yeast

1 to 2 tablespoons lemon juice

¼ cup (57 grams) Coconut Butter (page 33); if mixing by hand, soften butter by placing the container in a bowl of warm water

2 tablespoons diced herbs, such as basil, parsley, thyme, or green onion, plus a bit more for garnish

- Preheat the oven to 350°F. Prepare a Perfect Coconut Pie Crust and prebake for 10 minutes.

- In a large skillet over medium heat, place the coconut oil or bacon fat. Sauté the onions until they begin to soften, about 3 minutes. Add the zucchini, bacon, salt, and pepper, and sauté until they begin to soften, about 2 minutes.

- In a large mixing bowl, blender, or food processor, mix together the eggs, coconut milk, salt and pepper to taste, mustard, nutritional yeast, lemon juice, and coconut butter.

- Add the onion mixture and herbs to the eggs. Stir in by hand. Pour into the pie crust.

- Bake for 30 to 35 minutes, on a tray in case of leaks, until puffed and set. The quiche can be slightly wiggly in the center.

- Cool for 15 minutes. Garnish with chopped herbs, and serve.

Gluten-free	Dairy-free	Egg-free	Meat-free	Tree Nut-free	Vegan	Diabetic-friendly	Candida-friendly	High-protein	10 minutes or less
●	●			●		●	●		

QUICHE LORRAINE

The legendary quiche that forged France's culinary glory was originally made with eggs, heavy cream, and smoked bacon inside a brioche dough. Quiche Lorraine has since evolved, and, in this Paleo-adapted recipe, I tried to emulate the flavor of heavy cream and rich Emmentaler cheese, using hunt-and-gather ingredients. See tips for a perfect quiche, page 217. Quiche is easy to make ahead the night before, refrigerate, and bake in the morning. Look for meat that is non-GMO and sugar-free. Freeze leftovers wrapped in individual slices, defrost in the refrigerator overnight, and reheat in the oven for 20 minutes for a quick meal.

YIELD: One 9-inch quiche; serves four to six • **EQUIPMENT:** A blender or food processor is helpful but not required

1 recipe Perfect Coconut Pie Crust (page 46)
1 tablespoon coconut oil
½ cup finely chopped onion
½ cup natural prosciutto, or bacon, cooked and cut into ½-inch pieces
2 green onions, diced
5 large eggs at room temperature
1½ cups unsweetened full-fat coconut milk (page 13)

¼ teaspoon unprocessed salt
¼ teaspoon black pepper
⅛ teaspoon ground nutmeg
2 tablespoons nutritional yeast
1 tablespoon lemon juice
⅓ cup (75 grams) Coconut Butter (page 33); if mixing by hand, soften butter by placing the container in a bowl of warm water
⅛ teaspoon ground cayenne
1 tablespoon diced green onion for garnish

- Preheat the oven to 350°F. Prepare a Perfect Coconut Pie Crust in a 9-inch pie pan, and prebake for 10 minutes.

- In a medium skillet, heat the coconut oil until a drop of water sizzles when flicked on it. Add the onion and green onions. Sauté for 2 to 3 minutes until they begin to soften.

- Layer the meat, onion, and green onion in the bottom of the prebaked pie crust.

- In a blender, food processor, or large mixing bowl, mix the eggs, coconut milk, salt, pepper, nutmeg, nutritional yeast, lemon juice, coconut butter, and cayenne. Pour into the crust over the meat and vegetables.

- Bake for 30 to 35 minutes, on a tray in case of leaks, until the quiche is puffed and set. It can be slightly wiggly in the center. Cool for 15 minutes, garnish with the green onions, and serve.

Gluten-free	Dairy-free	Egg-free	Meat-free	Tree Nut-free	Vegan	Diabetic-friendly	Candida-friendly	High-protein	10 minutes or less
●	●			●		●	●		

SPICY CHIPOTLE SAUSAGE QUICHE

This is a zesty quiche with a vibrant Southwest flavor—and these flavors are heightened when you serve it with Cilantro Pesto (page 253) or Paleo Sour Cream (page 256). Quiche is easy to make ahead the night before and bake in the morning. See tips for a perfect quiche, page 217. Freeze leftovers in individually wrapped portions. Then defrost in the refrigerator overnight, and bake for about 20 minutes in the oven.

YIELD: One 9-inch quiche

1 recipe Perfect Coconut Pie Crust (page 46)
1 tablespoon coconut oil
1 garlic clove, diced
¾ cup chopped onion
8 ounces Spicy Chorizo (page 237), or your favorite bulk sausage
1½ teaspoons chili powder
¼ teaspoon pure chipotle powder

4 large eggs at room temperature
1 cup unsweetened full-fat coconut milk (page 13)
¼ teaspoon unprocessed salt
¼ teaspoon black pepper
2 tablespoons nutritional yeast
2 tablespoons lemon juice
2 green onions, diced
2 tomatoes, diced thinly

- Preheat the oven to 350°F. Prepare a Perfect Coconut Pie Crust in a 9-inch pie pan, and prebake for 10 minutes.

- In a large skillet over medium heat, place the oil. Sauté the garlic and onion for 1 to 2 minutes. Add the sausage, chili powder, and chipotle powder. Heat for 3 to 4 minutes until the sausage is barely cooked. Put the mixture in the bottom of the baked pie crust.

- In a medium mixing bowl, blender, or food processor, mix together the eggs, coconut milk, salt, pepper, nutritional yeast, and lemon juice. Add green onions and tomatoes, and stir by hand. Pour into the crust over the meat and vegetables.

- Bake for 30 to 35 minutes, on a tray in case of leaks, until the quiche is puffed and set. It can be slightly wiggly in the center. Cool for 15 minutes and serve.

Gluten-free	Dairy-free	Egg-free	Meat-free	Tree Nut–free	Vegan	Diabetic-friendly	Candida-friendly	High-protein	10 minutes or less
●	●			●		●	●		

SPINACH AND FETA QUICHE

This Mediterranean-style quiche makes a hearty breakfast, with spinach, herbs, and feta cheese that melt and blend in every bite. If you don't like spinach you could substitute broccoli, leek, or kale. See tips for a perfect quiche, page 217. Quiche is easy to make ahead the night before, refrigerate, and bake in the morning. Leftover slices of quiche can be frozen in an air-tight container for another day when you need a quick, nutritious breakfast.

YIELD: Serves six

1 recipe Perfect Coconut Pie Crust (page 46)
2 tablespoons coconut or olive oil
½ medium onion, diced
2 cloves chopped garlic (optional)
3 cups coarsely chopped raw baby spinach
⅔ cup Paleo Feta Cheese (page 44), or grass-fed goat cheese in small chunks

4 large eggs at room temperature
½ cup unsweetened full-fat coconut milk (page 13)
½ teaspoon unprocessed salt, or to taste
¼ teaspoon black pepper
¼ cup fresh chopped herbs, such as oregano, basil, tarragon or thyme, or use 1 tablespoon dried herbs
1 tomato, sliced thinly

- Preheat the oven to 350°F. Prepare a Perfect Coconut Pie Crust in a 9-inch pie pan and prebake for 10 minutes.

- In a large skillet over medium heat, place the oil. Sauté the onion and garlic until they begin to soften, about 2 minutes. Add the spinach and cook very briefly for 30 seconds just to wilt. Put the spinach mixture into the bottom of the baked pie shell and sprinkle feta cheese on top.

- In a large mixing bowl, blender, or food processor, mix together the eggs, coconut milk, salt, and pepper. Add the herbs and stir by hand. Pour the egg mixture into the pie shell over the vegetables, and stir it a bit to mix into the spinach. Top with tomato slices.

- Bake for 30 to 35 minutes, on a tray in case of leaks, until the quiche is puffed and set. It can be slightly wiggly in the center. Cool for 15 minutes and serve.

Gluten-free	Dairy-free	Egg-free	Meat-free	Tree Nut-free	Vegan	Diabetic-friendly	Candida-friendly	High-protein	10 minutes or less
●	●		●	●		●	●		

WILD SALMON LEEK QUICHE, OR MINI QUICHES

Full-bodied flavor is the theme of the day with this succulent combination of wild salmon, leeks, and mushrooms. Look for wild Alaskan salmon, which is higher in omega-3 fatty acids and protein, with fewer toxins—a better value for the nutrition even though it costs a bit more. The leeks can be substituted with onions or shallots. Use your favorite mushrooms, such as button, crimini, or shiitake. See tips for a perfect quiche, page 217. You can prep it in the evening, bake it in the morning, and freeze the leftovers. If you don't have time to make the crust, just pour the filling into greased muffin tins for mini quiches—a quick meal on the go.

YIELD: One 9-inch quiche or twelve to fourteen crustless mini quiches • **EQUIPMENT:** A blender or food processor is helpful but not required

1 recipe Perfect Coconut Pie Crust (page 46)
1 tablespoon coconut oil
2 cups leeks, diced
½ cup mushrooms, sliced (optional)
8 ounces cooked wild salmon, in small pieces
4 large eggs at room temperature
¾ cup unsweetened full-fat coconut milk (page 13)
¼ teaspoon unprocessed salt
¼ teaspoon black pepper
⅛ teaspoon ground nutmeg
2 tablespoons nutritional yeast
1 tablespoon lemon juice
¼ cup (57 grams) Coconut Butter (page 33); if mixing by hand, soften butter by placing the container in a bowl of warm water
1 tablespoon diced parsley or herbs, plus a bit more for garnish

- Preheat the oven to 350°F. Prepare a Perfect Coconut Pie Crust and prebake for 10 minutes. If you're making mini quiches, grease and flour a 12-cup muffin tin with coconut oil and coconut flour.

- In a large skillet over medium heat, place the oil. Sauté the leeks until they begin to soften, about 3 minutes. Add the mushrooms, salt and pepper to taste, and sauté briefly, about 2 minutes.

continues

continued

- Layer leeks, mushrooms, and salmon in the bottom of the prebaked pie crust or muffin cups.

- In a large mixing bowl, blender, or food processor, mix together the eggs, coconut milk, salt, pepper, nutmeg, nutritional yeast, lemon juice, and coconut butter. Stir in parsley. Pour over the leeks, mushrooms, and salmon.

- Bake for 30 to 35 minutes, on a tray in case of spills. Or bake muffins for 22 to 28 minutes, until the custard is golden, puffed, and set. The quiche can be slightly wiggly in the center.

- Cool for 15 minutes. Garnish with parsley or herbs.

Gluten-free	Dairy-free	Egg-free	Meat-free	Tree Nut–free	Vegan	Diabetic-friendly	Candida-friendly	High-protein	10 minutes or less
●	●			●		●	●		

10

MEATS AND
OTHER WILD BREAKFASTS

"A good meal soothes the soul as it regenerates the body."
—Frederick W. Hackwood

Proteins are very important for our health and well-being—and a high-protein breakfast will provide a firm foundation for your day. With its high-protein content, meat provides a balanced blood sugar level throughout the day. A breakfast of sugar and other simple carbs can give you a quick lift, but those carbs are quickly burned up, and that energetic feeling can't last. Soon you're hungry again and looking for the next sugar fix. Meat can help provide stable energy levels, improved mental focus, and fewer cravings all day.

When you're shopping for meat, look for grass-fed, pastured meats, poultry, and wild-caught fish, all without added sugars or chemicals. This is the best way to avoid antibiotics, hormones, and poor-quality GMO feed. And it most closely emulates

the ancestral diet. It is important to specifically ask for meats that are grass-fed and not fed GMO-grains. Sometimes you can find these in your local healthy grocery. There are many online sources—check out the listings at eatwild.com, a directory of pastured-based farms.

It's a good idea to vary your types of protein, in order to benefit from the different nutritional profiles of meats, as well as saving money on economical organ meats. A few possibilities to consider are grass-fed beef, organic chicken, and pastured organ meats such as liver and kidney.

This chapter includes a variety of meat-based breakfasts, including savory ethnic dishes, rich organ meats, and amazing homemade sausage. They're designed to be easy to make and tasty for the whole family.

227

BEEF FAJITAS WITH SPICY CHEESE SAUCE

Tender beef strips seasoned with cilantro and spices, served in a grain-free tortilla. And if your tortillas are made ahead, this takes just 10 minutes from start to finish. Try it with a side of Fermented Veggies (page 48). Freeze leftovers in BPA-free containers for another day.

YIELD: Serves four • **EQUIPMENT:** You'll need a blender for the sauce

¼ cup olive oil
1 tablespoon lemon juice
3 tablespoons diced cilantro
3 cloves garlic, diced
1½ teaspoons ground cumin
½ teaspoon chili powder
1 teaspoon unprocessed salt
1 teaspoon ground black pepper
2 (8 ounces each) boneless New York strip steaks, cut into thin strips
1 medium onion, sliced in half-moons
1 red bell pepper, sliced into strips
1 recipe Easy Burrito Wraps (page 76), Chia Corn Tortillas (page 73),
    or Plantain Tortillas (page 75)
1 cup of your favorite salsa
1 recipe Spicy Cheese Sauce (page 258)

- In a large mixing bowl, whisk together the olive oil, lemon juice, cilantro, garlic, cumin, chili powder, salt, and black pepper. Add the steak strips, onion, and bell pepper, stirring together to marinate. You can cook them right away, or marinate in the refrigerator overnight.

- Put the beef mixture into a large skillet over medium heat. Sauté for a few minutes until the beef is cooked through. Add a few tablespoons of filtered water if necessary to prevent sticking.

- Spoon into Paleo tortillas. Top with salsa and Spicy Cheese Sauce and serve.

Gluten-free	Dairy-free	Egg-free	Meat-free	Tree Nut-free	Vegan	Diabetic-friendly	Candida-friendly	High-protein	10 minutes or less
●	●	●		●		●	●	●	●

CHICKEN ADOBO ON TORTILLAS

Classic adobo sauce is super-easy to make in the blender. This recipe has the authentic sweet and spicy flavor, but without the sugar rush, to keep you on an even keel all morning. For a genuine adobo taste, look for chile molido, also called ground New Mexico chile, by Los Chileros, a national brand from Santa Fe. Their Chile Chipotle Powder is made from smoked jalapeño peppers with no additives or sweeteners. It's hot, so you don't need much. If you prepare the tortillas ahead and freeze, this is a snap to make—just blend the sauce and pour over chicken pieces for a quick and satisfying breakfast. Use the Easy Burrito Wraps (page 76), Plantain Tortillas (page 75), or Chia Corn Tortillas (page 73).

YIELD: 2 cups adobo; serves four

ADOBO SAUCE:
1 medium onion, in coarse chunks
2 cloves garlic, in chunks
1½ tablespoons apple cider vinegar
1 teaspoon unprocessed salt
Black pepper to taste
3 tablespoons coconut oil
About 1½ tablespoons sweetener to taste (see options on page 18)
½ teaspoon dried or fresh oregano
½ teaspoon dried or fresh thyme
½ teaspoon ground cumin
¼ teaspoon ground cinnamon
⅛ teaspoon ground allspice
A pinch of ground cloves
1 tablespoon chile molido mild, or chili powder
¼ teaspoon pure chile chipotle powder

FAJITAS:
½ pound cooked chicken meat, shredded or in ½-inch chunks
4 tortilla wraps, such as Easy Burrito Wraps (page 76), Chia Corn Tortillas (page 73), or Plantain Tortillas (page 75)
1 cup chopped greens, such as baby arugula or spinach

- In a small blender mix together the onion, garlic, vinegar, salt, pepper, oil, sweetener, herbs, cumin, cinnamon, allspice, cloves, chile molido, and chipotle powder. Blend well until completely liquefied.

- Pour the sauce into a large skillet over medium heat. Add the chicken meat and heat to boiling. Place the tortillas on a plate and add the chopped greens, topping with chicken in adobo sauce. Serve.

Gluten-free	Dairy-free	Egg-free	Meat-free	Tree Nut-free	Vegan	Diabetic-friendly	Candida-friendly	High-protein	10 minutes or less
●	●	●		●		●	●	●	●

CHICKEN LIVERS WITH BACON ON TOAST

Chicken livers are highly nutritious, easy to prepare, and economical. If you're not a fan of liver, keep reading. Homemade Bacon Bits (page 42), garlic, and lemon juice soften the flavor of the liver and give this dish an irresistible zing. Look for pastured livers and non-GMO, sugar-free bacon when possible. If you're able to make ahead and freeze the bread, this is a super-quick breakfast. Any toasted bread in this book will work—my favorites are the Fluffy Almond Butter Bread (page 54) and Fluffy White Bread (page 55).

YIELD: Serves two

1 tablespoon coconut oil
1 medium onion, chopped
1 clove garlic, crushed or diced
8 ounces chicken livers
Unprocessed salt and black pepper to taste
2 teaspoons arrowroot flour
A few tablespoons broth or filtered water, if necessary
1 tablespoon chopped parsley
1 tablespoon lemon juice
¼ cup Homemade Bacon Bits (page 42),
    or 3 slices cooked bacon, in small pieces (optional)
A pinch of cayenne
4 slices toasted Paleo bread

- In a skillet, melt the coconut oil over medium heat. Sauté the onion and garlic briefly, about 2 minutes.

- Add the chicken livers and salt and pepper. Use a fine gauge strainer to sprinkle arrowroot on top. Stir it in and cook until the chicken livers are firm and lightly browned, about 4 minutes. Add a few tablespoons of filtered water to make a gravy and keep the chicken livers from sticking to the pan.

- Add the parsley, lemon juice, bacon, and cayenne. Reduce the heat, cover, and simmer gently for 5 minutes or so, adding more liquid if necessary. Serve on toast.

Gluten-free	Dairy-free	Egg-free	Meat-free	Tree Nut-free	Vegan	Diabetic-friendly	Candida-friendly	High-protein	10 minutes or less
●	●	●		●		●	●	●	●

EASY LIVER PÂTÉ

Liver is one of Nature's most potent superfoods. It contains more nutrients, gram for gram, than any other food. Liver is an excellent source of protein, is high in all the B vitamins, vitamin A, CoQ10, folic acid, and iron. This pâté tastes rich and creamy, much like traditional pâté de foi gras. The main difference is that you can make it in 15 minutes or less! I wanted a way to prepare liver with minimal cooking for a soft texture, and to preserve nutrients. This came out velvety smooth and delectable. Refrigerate the pate up to 3 days. Or freeze in ice cube trays overnight; then transfer cubes to a resealable freezer bag, to enjoy a little at a time. Just one cube makes an economical, high-nutrition breakfast. Tastes wonderful on toasted English Muffins (page 67).

YIELD: 2 cups • **EQUIPMENT:** A food processor or any blender

1 pound pasture-fed liver (chicken, duck, beef, etc.)
2 tablespoons coconut oil
2 cloves garlic
¼ cup minced onions or shallots
1 tablespoon lemon juice
¼ cup full-fat coconut milk (page 13)
⅛ teaspoon ground allspice

2 teaspoons dried rosemary
¼ teaspoon ground mustard
1 teaspoon chopped fresh thyme (optional)
½ cup melted coconut oil (place the container in a bowl of warm water) or melted bacon fat.
¼ teaspoon unprocessed salt, or more to taste
⅛ teaspoon ground black pepper

- Trim the liver to remove any spots and cut into coarse 1-inch chunks.

- Melt the coconut oil over medium heat in a skillet. Add the garlic and onions and sauté briefly until they begin to soften, about 1 minute. Add the liver and sauté briefly until it is just barely cooked through, but not tough.

- Place the mixture in a blender or food processor. Add the lemon juice, coconut milk, and seasonings. Cover and process until the liver is a smooth paste. This will be about 30 seconds in a super-blender. In a regular blender or food processor it will take several minutes, and it helps to open the machine, stir the mixture away from the sides, and process again a few times.

- Add the oil, salt, and pepper. Process until the mixture is very smooth. Adjust the seasoning.

- Pour into a serving bowl, storage container, or ice cube trays. Chill to firm up even more. Make sure the containers are completely covered with plastic wrap directly on the pâté to prevent oxidation.

Gluten-free	Dairy-free	Egg-free	Meat-free	Tree Nut-free	Vegan	Diabetic-friendly	Candida-friendly	High-protein	10 minutes or less
●	●	●		●		●	●	●	●

SAUTÉED KIDNEY WITH ONIONS AND LEMON

You'll be amazed at the delicate flavor of this easy Italian recipe called *Rognoni trifolati con cipolla e limone*. When kidneys are quickly sautéed in onion, garlic, and lemon, it softens the distinctive kidney flavor and creates delicious gravy. Organ meats are nutritional powerhouses, and especially healthy if you're feeling chronically tired. Look for grass-fed, grass-finished organ meats (see Resources—Buying Guide on page 271). This is wonderful served over toasted bread, such as Almond Sandwich Bread (page 53) or Fluffy White Bread (page 55). Freeze leftovers in BPA-free containers.

YIELD: Serves two

¾ pound beef kidney
1 teaspoon apple cider vinegar
2 tablespoons olive oil
1 medium onion, sliced
1 clove garlic, chopped
Unprocessed salt and black pepper to taste
2 tablespoons coconut flour or arrowroot powder

1 green onion, chopped
2 tablespoons fresh parsley, chopped
Zest of 1 lemon
1 teaspoon lemon juice
2 teaspoons nutritional yeast
3 to 5 tablespoons filtered water or broth

- Remove fat and veins from the kidney with a paring knife and cut into bite-size pieces. Immerse the pieces in filtered water with the vinegar for 30 minutes or overnight, to clean and soften the flavor. Drain the pieces and pat them dry.

- In a large skillet, heat the oil over medium-high heat. Sauté the onion and garlic briefly, for about 2 minutes.

- Add the kidney pieces, salt, and pepper. Sprinkle with coconut flour. Stir in the water, green onion, parsley, lemon zest, lemon juice, and nutritional yeast.

- Sauté over high heat for 4 to 5 minutes, until the kidneys are just barely cooked through. Add a few tablespoons more water or broth if desired. Serve.

Gluten-free	Dairy-free	Egg-free	Meat-free	Tree Nut-free	Vegan	Diabetic-friendly	Candida-friendly	High-protein	10 minutes or less
●	●	●		●		●	●	●	

WILD SALMON CAKES WITH SOUR CREAM

Wild salmon creates a flavorful breakfast that's loaded with protein and omega-3 nutrition. These cakes are tasty with any wild fish such as sea bass, halibut, or true cod. You can bake these delectable morsels in the oven, or they also cook quicker and brown nicely in a skillet. Serve with a dollop of Paleo Sour Cream (page 256) and a side of Fermented Veggies (page 48). Freeze leftover cooked patties in an airtight container for another day.

YIELD: Five 2½-inch patties

10 ounces wild salmon
2 large eggs, pasture raised, organic
3 green onions, chopped
1 tablespoon lemon or lime juice
2 to 3 tablespoons fresh herbs, such as basil,
    parsley, cilantro, dill, tarragon,
¼ teaspoon unprocessed salt or to taste
¼ teaspoon black pepper
½ teaspoon ground mustard
½ cup almond meal
2 tablespoons coconut oil for cooking

- To cook the salmon, place the fillets skin-down in a large skillet with ¼ inch filtered water. Cover and bring to a gentle boil over low heat to steam gently for 3 to 4 minutes. Add a bit more water if it boils dry. When the salmon turns a light color, put it on a plate to cool for 10 minutes, remove the skin and bones, dice, and set aside.

- In a medium mixing bowl, whisk the eggs. Stir in the green onions, lemon juice, herbs, salt, pepper, mustard, and almond meal. Add the salmon and stir with a spatula to combine.

- Heat the oil in a large skillet over medium heat. When a drop of water flicked onto the pan sizzles, it's ready. Use a ⅓ cup measure to make five patties with your hands. Drop them into the hot skillet. Cook for 4 to 5 minutes on each side.

- If you're baking them, bake at 350°F on a parchment-covered baking tray for a total of 20 minutes, 10 minutes on each side. Serve!

Gluten-free	Dairy-free	Egg-free	Meat-free	Tree Nut-free	Vegan	Diabetic-friendly	Candida-friendly	High-protein	10 minutes or less
●	●					●	●	●	

WILD SALMON WITH GARLICKY GREENS

Here's a savory, satisfying breakfast you can make in 5 minutes flat. While the salmon steams for 4 minutes, sauté the greens, and serve! You can use your favorite wild fish, such as sea bass, halibut, or true cod. Any leafy greens will work, such as nutrient-dense kale, turnip greens, beet tops, chard, rapini greens, sunflower sprouts, etc. For the highest nutrition, minerals, and omega-3's, look for wild-caught fish.

YIELD: Serves two

½ pound fresh wild salmon
Unprocessed salt and black pepper to taste
2 tablespoons coconut oil or olive oil
3 to 5 cloves garlic, crushed or diced
4 handfuls greens, coarsely chopped into 2-inch squares
2 to 3 tablespoons nutritional yeast
2 to 3 tablespoons lemon juice
⅛ teaspoon unprocessed salt

- To cook the salmon, place the fillet in a small skillet over medium heat with ¼ inch filtered water, salt, and pepper. Bring to a boil, cover, and turn down to a very low simmer for about 4 minutes to steam. When the salmon is lighter in color and barely cooked, cool, remove the skin and bones, and set aside.

- Heat the oil in a large skillet over medium heat. Sauté the garlic briefly until it sizzles, but do not allow it to brown (it turns bitter), about 1 minute. Add the greens and toss to distribute the garlic evenly into the leaves. Sauté for 3 to 4 minutes. Then add 2 tablespoons of water, cover, and steam for 1 to 3 minutes or until the greens are tender.

- Stir in the nutritional yeast, lemon juice, and additional salt, if desired. Plate the greens and top with the salmon. Enjoy!

Gluten-free	Dairy-free	Egg-free	Meat-free	Tree Nut-free	Vegan	Diabetic-friendly	Candida-friendly	High-protein	10 minutes or less
●	●	●		●		●	●	●	●

HOMEMADE BREAKFAST SAUSAGE

This simple homemade sausage is so easy you'll never want to eat store-bought sausage again. It tastes slightly sweet with a blend of traditional spices and a hint of maple. While the recipe calls for pork, it is also delicious with turkey, chicken, beef, lamb, and bison. This sausage is perfect for Biscuits and Gravy (page 176) or Breakfast Tacos (page 178). Wrap individually and freeze the raw patties so you can look forward to a nutritious breakfast any day.

YIELD: Four patties 2 to 3 inches in diameter

12 ounces ground pork
1 tablespoon chopped sage, or 1 teaspoon ground sage
¼ teaspoon ground nutmeg
1 teaspoon chopped fresh rosemary
 or ½ teaspoon crushed dried rosemary
½ teaspoon fennel seed, ground
¾ teaspoon unprocessed salt
½ teaspoon black pepper
1 clove garlic, crushed
½ teaspoon ground allspice
⅛ teaspoon maple flavor
1 teaspoon sweetener (see options on page 18)

- In a medium bowl, add all the ingredients and mix well with a rubber spatula or your hands.

- If you're making patties, with your hands, form four patties 2 to 3 inches round. Fry the patties on both sides in a nonstick pan over medium heat until completely cooked through and golden brown, about 4 to 5 minutes on each side.

- If you're preparing loose sausage, do not form the patties; fry in 1 tablespoon oil in a nonstick pan, breaking up the sausage into small pieces. Cook for 3 to 5 minutes or until no longer pink. Serve.

Gluten-free	Dairy-free	Egg-free	Meat-free	Tree Nut-free	Vegan	Diabetic-friendly	Candida-friendly	High-protein	10 minutes or less
●	●	●		●		●	●	●	

GREEN CHILE LAMB SAUSAGE

This traditional New Mexican sausage is mildly spicy with an irresistible Southwest flavor. The secret ingredients are smoked paprika and green chiles. Traditionally made with lamb, you can also try it with pork, beef, turkey, chicken, rabbit, etc. So easy to make, you can use this a hundred ways: fry it with scrambled eggs, serve patties on a bed of greens, or put it in Breakfast Burritos (page 177). It tastes amazing with Paleo Sour Cream (page 256) or Cilantro Pesto (page 253). Freeze the raw patties individually wrapped, defrost overnight, and cook for a super-quick breakfast.

YIELD: 1 pound bulk sausage or eight 2½-inch patties; serves four

1 pound ground lamb
1 teaspoon unprocessed salt
¼ teaspoon black pepper
4 garlic cloves, crushed or diced
2 teaspoons smoked paprika
½ teaspoon allspice
6 tablespoons chopped green chiles, well drained
   (half of a 4-ounce can, mild or spicy)
⅛ teaspoon red pepper flakes or cayenne powder
1 tablespoon apple cider vinegar
2 tablespoons diced cilantro

- In a medium bowl, mix all the ingredients well with a rubber spatula or your hands.

- If you're making patties, with your hands, form four patties 2 to 3 inches round. Fry the patties on both sides in a nonstick pan over medium heat until completely cooked through and golden brown, about 4 to 5 minutes on each side.

- If you're preparing loose sausage, do not form the patties; fry in 1 tablespoon oil in a nonstick pan, breaking up the sausage into small pieces. Cook for 3 to 5 minutes or until no longer pink. Serve.

Gluten-free	Dairy-free	Egg-free	Meat-free	Tree Nut-free	Vegan	Diabetic-friendly	Candida-friendly	High-protein	10 minutes or less
●	●	●		●		●	●	●	

SPICY CHORIZO

This zesty Mexican-style sausage is a flavorful addition to breakfasts with a Southwest flavor. You can use it so many ways: add it to sautéed veggies, use it to spice up scrambled eggs, or put it in a burrito. Chorizo is traditionally made with pork, however, it is tasty made with beef, turkey, chicken, or bison. Freeze the raw patties individually wrapped, and defrost them in the refrigerator overnight to add protein and spice to any breakfast. Use this for Spicy Chipotle Sausage Quiche (page 223).

YIELD: 1 pound bulk sausage or eight 2½-inch patties; serves four

1 pound ground pork
4 teaspoons chili powder or mild chile molido powder
1 teaspoon pure chipotle powder
1 tablespoon paprika
¼ teaspoon ground cinnamon
⅛ teaspoon ground cloves
½ teaspoon ground cumin
1 teaspoon unprocessed salt
½ teaspoon freshly ground black pepper
1 tablespoon diced fresh oregano, or ½ tablespoon dried oregano
4 cloves garlic, crushed
3 tablespoons apple cider vinegar
Brown Sweetener is optional, up to 1 tablespoon (see options on page 18)

- In a medium bowl, add all the ingredients and mix well with a rubber spatula or your hands.

- If you're making patties, with your hands, form four patties 2 to 3 inches round. Fry the patties on both sides in a nonstick pan over medium heat until completely cooked through and golden brown, about 4 to 5 minutes on each side.

- If you're preparing loose sausage, do not form the patties; fry in 1 tablespoon oil in a nonstick pan, breaking up the sausage into small pieces. Cook for 3 to 5 minutes or until no longer pink. Serve.

Gluten-free	Dairy-free	Egg-free	Meat-free	Tree Nut–free	Vegan	Diabetic-friendly	Candida-friendly	High-protein	10 minutes or less
●	●	●		●		●	●	●	

TURKEY SAUSAGE WITH APPLE AND SAGE

This mellow sausage tastes like Thanksgiving but is great any time of year. Your taste buds might be a little surprised when they first encounter the subtle flavors of sweet apple, earthy sage and aromatic fennel. I think they're a great combination. Make it in 10 minutes and use it in a hundred ways. Fry it loose and serve on toast, stir it into your eggs, add it to a casserole or stir-fry. These patties actually taste better the next day, making them perfect for reheating. If you don't have a food processor, no worries, just dice the apple very fine. Freeze raw patties wrapped individually for next week's breakfasts in a flash.

YIELD: 1 pound bulk sausage or eight 2½-inch patties; serves four • **EQUIPMENT:** Food processor

1 Granny Smith apple, cored, including the peel
2 tablespoons onion flakes
3 tablespoons diced fresh sage leaves, or ½ teaspoon sage powder
½ teaspoon fennel seeds, crushed, ground, or chopped

¾ teaspoon unprocessed salt
½ teaspoon fresh ground pepper
½ teaspoon ground allspice
1 pound ground turkey, chicken, pork, beef, lamb, bison, rabbit, or squirrel

- In a food processor or mixing bowl, add all the ingredients except the meat: apple, onion flakes, sage, fennel, salt, pepper, and allspice. Process well until the apple is mostly liquefied. Open the processor and stir the sides if necessary and mix again. Add the meat and process again until all the ingredients are well combined.

- If you're making patties, with your hands, form four patties 2 to 3 inches round. Fry the patties on both sides in a nonstick pan over medium heat until completely cooked through and golden brown, about 4 to 5 minutes on each side.

- If you're preparing loose sausage, do not form the patties; fry in 1 tablespoon oil in a nonstick pan, breaking up the sausage into small pieces. Cook for 3 to 5 minutes or until no longer pink.

Gluten-free	Dairy-free	Egg-free	Meat-free	Tree Nut-free	Vegan	Diabetic-friendly	Candida-friendly	High-protein	10 minutes or less
●	●	●		●		●	●	●	

ZESTY ITALIAN SAUSAGE

Mamma mia! Authentic Italian flavor with the perfect blend of fresh herbs and spices, this easy sausage is a great one to keep stocked in your freezer at all times. If you have a few patties on hand, breakfast is a snap. It's rich with spicy and subtle flavors of onion, garlic, and fennel seeds. So easy to make, you'll never want store-bought sausage again. This is traditionally made with pork, however it is also delicious with ground turkey, chicken, beef, lamb, or bison. Look for non-GMO grass-fed meat. Try it in the Open-Faced Focaccia with Sausage (page 179) or Mediterranean Eggs with Spinach and Sausage (page 205). Freeze the patties individually wrapped, for an easy, flavorful breakfast.

12 ounces ground pork

2 teaspoons apple cider vinegar

¾ teaspoon unprocessed salt

¾ teaspoon black pepper

2 cloves garlic, crushed

1 tablespoon onion flakes

¼ cup finely chopped herbs, such as basil, oregano, thyme, tarragon, or parsley

A pinch of cayenne, or ⅛ teaspoon red pepper flakes

½ teaspoon whole fennel seeds, crushed

½ teaspoon crushed anise seeds, or anise powder (optional)

Sweetener is optional, 0 to 2 teaspoons (see options on page 18)

1 tablespoon olive oil (optional), depending on the fat content of your pork

- In a medium bowl, mix all the ingredients together well with a firm rubber spatula or with your hands.

- If you're making patties, with your hands, form four patties 2 to 3 inches round. Fry the patties on both sides in a nonstick pan over medium heat until completely cooked through and golden brown, about 4 to 5 minutes on each side.

- If you're preparing loose sausage, do not form the patties; fry in 1 tablespoon oil in a nonstick pan, breaking up the sausage into small pieces. Cook for 3 to 5 minutes or until no longer pink. Serve.

Gluten-free	Dairy-free	Egg-free	Meat-free	Tree Nut-free	Vegan	Diabetic-friendly	Candida-friendly	High-protein	10 minutes or less
●	●	●		●		●	●	●	

11

SAUCES, TOPPINGS, AND JAMS

"Your diet is like a bank account.
Good food choices are good investments."
—Bethenny Frankel

The healthiest foods deserve the best condiments. I want you to enjoy every delightful taste, every texture, every combination of sauces, dips, and syrups humanly possible, all comprised of healthy, nutrient-dense food. It's all too easy to eat "mostly Paleo" and risk trashing your clean diet with store-bought sauces loaded with sugar and preservatives. Now you can skip the processed condiments in favor of these sauces. If you sweeten with the recommended sweeteners (page 18), you can drastically cut your sugar intake without sacrificing flavor or enjoyment.

We're talking vast differences in carbs and sugars in these recipes. For example, let's look at the sugar content in a few recipes. Two tablespoons of conventional blueberry jam contain 21 grams of sugars.

Compare that to 2 tablespoons of this Blueberry Chia Jam (page 244) with just 2 grams of sugars. Hot caramel sauce tastes delightful on Pecan Waffles (page 127). Which sauce do you choose? Just ¼ cup of conventional caramel sauce contains 24 grams of sugars. However the same amount of Paleo Hot Caramel Sauce (page 248) has less than 1 gram of sugars.

It's not just the sweeter condiments, either. Ketchup is a must for my Wild Salmon Cauliflower Hash (page 174). Should I use 2 tablespoons of Heinz ketchup with 8 grams of sugars? Probably not, since the same amount of Homemade Ketchup (page 255) has just 1.4 grams sugars.

You deserve the real food flavors in these healthy condiments. Blend up a quick Berrylicious Sauce (page 243) for pancakes or waffles. Try Blueberry Chia Jam (page 244) on your toast. Taste savory classics like Hollandaise Sauce (page 254) and Spicy Cheese Sauce (page 258) on flatbread. Add versatile condiments like Avocado Pesto (page 252) and Cilantro Pesto (page 253) to your eggs or breakfast tacos. Freeze leftover sauces and jams overnight in an ice cube tray enclosed in a plastic bag to avoid freezer flavors. Then transfer the cubes to a resealable bag for future use.

These healthy sauces are intended to help you cut down on sugar consumption with no loss in flavor, so you can enjoy a productive day of mental clarity and balanced metabolism.

BERRYLICIOUS SAUCE

This high-antioxidant sauce is both easy and scrumptious—a perfect match for pancakes, waffles, or French toast. You can't beat the flavor of simple blended berries, and their natural pectin, which thickens the sauce naturally. Use any low-sugar berry, such as blueberry, raspberry, gooseberry, elderberry, etc., for a luscious, low-carb sauce. Blend it raw to conserve all the nutrients; if you prefer to serve it warm, heat briefly in a saucepan. Freeze leftover sauce in an ice cube tray overnight, then store cubes in a freezer bag for up to 6 weeks. Pull out a few cubes at a time to pour over pancakes or spread on your favorite toast.

YIELD: 1¼ cups sauce • **EQUIPMENT:** Any blender

2 cups (10 ounces) fresh tart berries, or frozen, thawed, and well drained
1 tablespoon lemon lime juice
A dash of vanilla
About 6 tablespoons sweetener to taste (see options on page 18)

- Place all the ingredients in any blender. Blend until very smooth.
- If you wish to remove the seeds, strain the sauce through a medium gauge strainer into a serving bowl.
- Pour over pancakes and enjoy!

VARIATION: Blackberry Sauce
Follow the recipe above, using 2 cups of blackberries instead of tart berries.

Gluten-free	Dairy-free	Egg-free	Meat-free	Tree Nut–free	Vegan	Diabetic-friendly	Candida-friendly	High-protein	10 minutes or less
●	●	●	●	●	●	●	●		●

BLUEBERRY CHIA JAM

Blended blueberries with chia seeds is the best jam in the world. Even better, you can enjoy it in minutes. This thick, low-sugar jam, tastes great on toasted Fluffy Almond Butter Bread (page 54) or English Muffins (page 67). Freeze leftover jam in an ice cube tray overnight, then store cubes in a freezer bag for up to 6 weeks, so you can pull out a cube at a time.

YIELD: ¾ cup jam • **EQUIPMENT:** Small blender or food processor

1 cup blueberries, fresh, or frozen, thawed, and very well drained
1½ teaspoons vanilla
1 teaspoon lemon zest
2 teaspoons lemon juice
Sweetener is optional, 0 to 2 tablespoons (see options on page 18)
1½ tablespoons whole black chia seeds

- In a food processor or small blender, mix the blueberries, vanilla, zest, lemon juice, and sweetener until smooth and liquefied.

- Add the chia seeds and process again. Let the jam sit in the machine for 10 minutes to thicken. Then process again until it is as smooth as possible. Serve.

Gluten-free	Dairy-free	Egg-free	Meat-free	Tree Nut–free	Vegan	Diabetic-friendly	Candida-friendly	High-protein	10 minutes or less
●	●	●	●	●	●	●	●		●

ORANGE MARMALADE

I think of oranges as pure concentrated sunshine. This homemade marmalade offers a taste of a bright morning—and it takes just a few minutes to make. For a spread that's easy on your blood sugar, use a zero-carb sweetener—see options (page 18). The best oranges for marmalade are organic Valencia, because they have thin skins, less bitter white pulp, and fewer toxins. Slather this on Fluffy Almond Butter Bread (page 53), English Muffins (page 67), Pecan Waffles (page 127), or just about anything. Refrigerate for a week or more. Freeze leftover marmalade in an ice cube tray overnight, then store cubes in a freezer bag for up to 6 weeks, for a taste of sunshine when you need it.

YIELD: 1 cup marmalade • **EQUIPMENT:** Food processor or super-blender such as a Vitamix or Blendtec

3 organic oranges
½ organic lemon (Meyer, if available)
2 to 4 tablespoons filtered water
About ¾ cup sweetener to taste (see options on page 18)

- Slice oranges and lemon as thin as possible, keeping the peel intact but removing seeds as you go. A mandoline slicer is easy, or you can quickly do it by hand.

- Stack half of the orange slices, cut them into ½-inch pieces, and set aside.

- Put the remaining slices in a food processor or super-blender. Add water and process until the peel is mush.

- Put all the fruit in a small saucepan, including the pieces set aside. Add sweetener and bring slowly to a gentle boil for 15 to 20 minutes uncovered, stirring frequently, until the mixture is quite thick.

- Remove the pan from heat, and allow the mixture to set for 30 minutes. Serve.

Gluten-free	Dairy-free	Egg-free	Meat-free	Tree Nut-free	Vegan	Diabetic-friendly	Candida-friendly	High-protein	10 minutes or less
●	●	●	●	●	●	●	●		

MAPLE FLAVOR SYRUP

Whether it's Blueberry Pancakes (page 117) or Sour Cream Waffles (page 128), this is my go-to syrup for all griddle breakfasts. It's very easy to make, just heat and serve. Contemporary maple syrup is a high-carb, refined sweetener that our Paleo ancestors never knew. It takes 55 gallons of raw maple sap to produce 1 gallon of refined maple syrup. Honey is a better alternative, although high in carbs. See all the sweetener options (page 18)—any of them will work, and the flavor will depend on your choice. Store this syrup in the refrigerator for up to 3 days.

YIELD: ¾ cup

½ cup boiling filtered water
About 1½ cups sweetener to taste (See options on page 18.
   I suggest at least half brown sweetener for a richer flavor.)
2 teaspoons vanilla
¼ teaspoon maple flavor
A pinch of ground cinnamon
1 tablespoon coconut oil
A pinch of unprocessed salt

- In a small saucepan, whisk together all the ingredients. Bring to a boil for just a brief moment. Then remove from heat and pour into a serving pitcher. Serve warm.

VARIATIONS:

Maple Pecan Syrup
Follow the recipe above. In the final step, stir in ¼ teaspoon more cinnamon and ¾ cup finely chopped pecans. While it's tantalizing with any of the waffle and pancake recipes, it's especially delightful on Apple Bread Pudding (page 162).

Orange Maple Syrup
Follow the main recipe above. Zest one orange into a bowl. Then juice the orange into the bowl. Stir into the warm syrup and serve. Try it on Traditional Plantain Pancakes (page 119).

Gluten-free	Dairy-free	Egg-free	Meat-free	Tree Nut–free	Vegan	Diabetic-friendly	Candida-friendly	High-protein	10 minutes or less
●	●	●	●	●	●	●	●		●

GINGER CARDAMOM SYRUP

When you're in the mood for a heavenly syrup that's far beyond everyday maple, whip up this exotic mélange. Ginger and cardamom add an aromatic zing that's refreshing, hot, and peppery, sort of like warm spicy chai on your pancakes or waffles. It tastes delightful on Apple Fritters (page 135) or Cinnamon Swirl French Toast (page 131). Store leftover syrup in the refrigerator for up to 3 days.

YIELD: 1½ cups

¾ cup filtered water
About 1½ cups sweetener to taste (See options on page 18.
    I like half white, half brown in this recipe.)
⅛ teaspoon unprocessed salt
1 teaspoon vanilla
1-inch piece of fresh ginger root, peeled and diced,
    or ¼ teaspoon ground ginger
3 pods cardamom, crushed, or ¼ teaspoon ground cardamom
½ teaspoon ground cinnamon

- Mix all the ingredients in a saucepan.

- Heat to boiling briefly, stirring constantly. Let it simmer slowly for 3 to 5 minutes while the flavors infuse.

- Strain into a serving pitcher. Serve warm.

Gluten-free	Dairy-free	Egg-free	Meat-free	Tree Nut-free	Vegan	Diabetic-friendly	Candida-friendly	High-protein	10 minutes or less
●	●	●	●	●	●	●	●		●

HOT CARAMEL SAUCE

Traditional caramel sauce is creamy, dreamy, and oh so thick, made with heavy cream, sugar, and butter. This Paleo adaptation takes 5 minutes, and it's just as dreamy and creamy, something like salted caramel. The sauce tastes mouthwatering on Pecan Waffles (page 127) and Cinnamon Apple Sour Cream Coffeecake (page 153). Freeze leftovers in an ice cube tray overnight, then put cubes in a freezer bag for up to 6 weeks. Or store in the refrigerator for up to 3 days, and then heat gently on the stove.

YIELD: 1¼ cups

About 1¼ cups sweetener to taste (See options on page 18.
   For a rich caramel flavor, I suggest half brown sweetener.)
⅛ teaspoon unprocessed salt
1 teaspoon arrowroot flour
¾ cup unsweetened coconut milk (page 35) or nut milk (page 36)
1 teaspoon vanilla
¼ teaspoon maple flavor
1 tablespoon coconut oil

- In a small saucepan, whisk together the sweetener, salt, and arrowroot.

- Add milk and stir over medium heat until the sweetener dissolves.

- Add vanilla, maple, and coconut oil. Heat to boiling for a brief moment, then immediately turn way down to simmer, stirring constantly. The arrowroot will begin to thicken in about 1 to 2 minutes.

- Pour into a small serving pitcher or bowl. Allow it to cool and it will thicken a bit more. Enjoy!

Gluten-free	Dairy-free	Egg-free	Meat-free	Tree Nut–free	Vegan	Diabetic-friendly	Candida-friendly	High-protein	10 minutes or less
●	●	●	●	●	●	●	●		●

COCONUT CREAM TOPPING

This coconut cream topping beats any dairy variety, hands-down. You can make it in 1 minute, using full-fat canned coconut milk. It's tastier and healthier than real dairy cream. The key is using thick, full-fat coconut milk (not "lite"); keep a can in the refrigerator and you can have this topping in no time at all. It's perfect for Fruit with Coconut Cream Topping (page 90), Cinnamon Swirl French Toast (page 131), or your next inspired creation. Store in the refrigerator for up to 3 days.

YIELD: ⅔ cup

1 (14-ounce) can thick, full-fat unsweetened coconut milk (page 13)
About 1½ tablespoons sweetener to taste (see options on page 18)
1 teaspoon vanilla

- Chill the coconut milk in the can for 8 hours or overnight, until it thickens into a lovely cream. (Better yet, keep a can in the fridge at all times!)
- Open the can and poke a hole in the top cream with a spoon. Pour off the thin milk from the bottom to use in something else. Whisk until smooth. Stir in the sweetener and vanilla until smooth. Serve.

Tip: Occasionally this recipe comes out a bit lumpy, depending on the coconut milk. To make it perfectly smooth, you can blend it briefly with an immersion blender.

Gluten-free	Dairy-free	Egg-free	Meat-free	Tree Nut–free	Vegan	Diabetic-friendly	Candida-friendly	High-protein	10 minutes or less
●	●	●	●	●	●	●	●		●

CHIPOTLE BUTTER

Chile and chipotle powders combine with creamy honey butter for a spicy Southwest flavor. You can add garlic for an extra kick or leave it out for a bit of a mellower flavor. It tastes amazing on Bacon Chili Cornbread (page 71) or Chili Cheese Biscuits (page 69). Look for Chile Chipotle Powder by Los Chileros. It's pure smoked jalapeños, so go easy! Store in the refrigerator for 1 week, or freeze in ice cube trays overnight; then transfer to a resealable bag for later use.

YIELD: ⅓ cup

⅓ cup (75 grams) Coconut Butter (page 33), softened
   (place the container in a bowl of warm water)
2 teaspoons raw honey or 1 tablespoon zero-carb sweetener
   (see page 18 for options)
¼ teaspoon chili powder
A pinch of pure chipotle powder
2 teaspoons lemon or lime juice
½ teaspoon unprocessed salt
Black pepper to taste
1 small clove garlic, crushed (optional)

• In a small bowl, whisk together all the ingredients. Serve at room temperature.

Gluten-free	Dairy-free	Egg-free	Meat-free	Tree Nut-free	Vegan	Diabetic-friendly	Candida-friendly	High-protein	10 minutes or less
●	●	●	●	●					●

ORANGE HONEY BUTTER

This is a delightful blend of sweet orange and creamy coconut butter. Stir it together in moments for a taste of sunshine on your Sour Cream Waffles (page 128), Sweet Potato Popovers (page 167), or toasted bread. Store in the refrigerator for a week. Or freeze leftovers in an ice cube tray overnight, then store cubes in a freezer bag for up to 3 months, so you can pull out a few cubes at a time.

YIELD: ¾ cup

Zest of 1 orange
Juice of 1 orange (see Tip below)
½ teaspoon vanilla
¼ cup (57 grams) Coconut Butter (page 33), softened
   (place the container in a bowl of warm water)
A dash of ground cinnamon
2 pinches of unprocessed salt
Raw honey: about 2 tablespoons, or 3 tablespoons
   zero-carb sweetener (see options on page 18)

- Use a small blender to blend all the ingredients until smooth, or just stir together with a spoon and serve. Chill to harden.

Tip: To prepare the orange, first zest it. If you're using a blender, cut away the bitter white pith with a small serrated knife. Then slice, seed it, and place the slices in the blender. If you're mixing by hand, there's no need to cut away the pith. Just cut it in half and juice with a citrus reamer.

Gluten-free	Dairy-free	Egg-free	Meat-free	Tree Nut–free	Vegan	Diabetic-friendly	Candida-friendly	High-protein	10 minutes or less
●	●	●	●	●					●

AVOCADO PESTO

This super-easy avocado spread has a Parmesan cheese flavor with a hint of garlic. If you're going easy on garlic, you can omit that, and it will still be yummy. Use this on sandwiches like green mayo, as a savory spread on Focaccia Flat Bread (page 77), as a dip for veggies, or as a topping for hash. It's scrumptious on the Personal Pizza for One (page 180). Store in the refrigerator for up to 3 days.

YIELD: 1 cup • **EQUIPMENT:** A food processor is helpful but not required

1 ripe avocado, pitted, and peeled (if mixing by hand, mashed)
2 tablespoons lemon juice
2 tablespoons olive oil
¼ cup fresh basil leaves, diced
1 clove garlic, pressed
2 teaspoons nutritional yeast
¼ teaspoon unprocessed salt

- In a food processor or mixing bowl, place all the ingredients. Mix well until smooth and creamy.

Tip: If you're not serving this immediately, save the avocado seed. Place the seed on top of the pesto in the serving bowl until you're ready to serve. It will help to keep the avocado from turning brown.

Gluten-free	Dairy-free	Egg-free	Meat-free	Tree Nut-free	Vegan	Diabetic-friendly	Candida-friendly	High-protein	10 minutes or less
●	●	●	●	●	●	●	●		●

CILANTRO PESTO

Coconut butter provides richness to this easy blended pesto. It adds a spicy Southwest flavor to eggs, focaccia, hash, or veggies. Bright green in color, it's very tasty on Breakfast Tacos (page 178), Bacon-Wrapped Eggs (page 198), or Breakfast Burritos (page 177). Store in the refrigerator for up to 3 days.

YIELD: 1¼ cups • **EQUIPMENT:** Small blender or food processor

3 tablespoons olive oil
2 tablespoons lemon juice
1 large clove garlic
¼ teaspoon unprocessed salt
1 tablespoon nutritional yeast
½ teaspoon chili powder
¼ cup (57 grams) Coconut Butter (page 33);
   softened (place the container in a bowl of warm water)
1 full cup fresh cilantro including stems, packed tight
2 tablespoons filtered water, if necessary to thin

- In any blender, mix together the olive oil, lemon juice, garlic, salt, nutritional yeast, chili powder, and coconut butter. Blend well until smooth. Add the cilantro last and blend well again. Thin with a tiny bit of water if necessary to blend. Pour into a small pitcher, and serve.

Gluten-free	Dairy-free	Egg-free	Meat-free	Tree Nut-free	Vegan	Diabetic-friendly	Candida-friendly	High-protein	10 minutes or less
●	●	●	●	●	●	●	●		●

HOLLANDAISE SAUCE

Traditional hollandaise is made with egg yolks, melted butter, and lemon juice. This easy hollandaise is egg- and dairy-free, using coconut as a base. It tastes especially wonderful on Eggs Benedict (page 208) and Wild Salmon Cakes (page 233). Use as a mayo substitute on sandwiches, omelets, and vegetables. Unrefined red palm oil is optional and gives it a beautiful golden color. For best success, have all ingredients near room temperature, neither cold nor hot. Freeze leftover sauce in a BPA-free container. Or freeze in an ice cube tray overnight, then store cubes in a freezer bag for up to 3 months. Or store in the refrigerator for 3 days. Allow several hours for it to warm up to room temperature to be pourable.

YIELD: ¾ cup sauce • **EQUIPMENT:** Small blender or immersion blender

2 tablespoons fresh lemon juice
½ teaspoon unprocessed salt
4 tablespoons (57 grams) Coconut Butter (page 33);
    softened (place the container in a bowl of warm water)
A pinch of ground white or black pepper
A pinch of cayenne
1 teaspoon nutritional yeast
½ cup coconut oil, gently melted but not hot
    (put the jar in a bowl of lukewarm water)
½ tablespoon red palm oil (optional) for a beautiful golden color

- In a small blender or immersion blender, mix together the lemon juice, salt, coconut butter, pepper, cayenne, and nutritional yeast. Blend until smooth. Add the coconut oil slowly in a stream while blending, until smooth and creamy. Add the red palm oil last, if using, and blend again. The thickness of the sauce will depend on the temperature in your kitchen. On a warm day it will be runny, and in cool weather it will be thicker. You can control this by putting it in a warm spot or chilling it briefly, but do not subject the oil to extreme temperature changes or it may separate. Pour into a serving pitcher.

Gluten-free	Dairy-free	Egg-free	Meat-free	Tree Nut–free	Vegan	Diabetic-friendly	Candida-friendly	High-protein	10 minutes or less
●	●	●	●	●	●	●	●		●

HOMEMADE KETCHUP

Homemade ketchup is so easy and tasty, you'll never want store-bought again. Spicy, tart, and sweet all at the same time, you'll love it on everything! Try it on Sweet Potato Tots (page 185) or Sweet Potato Hash with Turkey Apple Sausage (page 170). It's quick to make in the blender, then simmer, and it's ready to enjoy. Look for a good quality tomato puree in a glass jar. Or you can buy crushed tomatoes—in this case, strain them in a sieve and press with a spatula to remove the excess liquid, otherwise your ketchup may be thin. Refrigerate in a glass jar for a week. Freeze leftover ketchup in an ice cube tray overnight, then store cubes in a freezer bag for up to 6 weeks, so you can pull out a cube at a time.

YIELD: 1½ cups

1½ cups tomato puree, or crushed tomatoes, well drained and pressed
About ¼ cup sweetener to taste (see options on page 18)
3 tablespoons apple cider vinegar
¼ teaspoon ground mustard
½ teaspoon unprocessed salt
1 small clove garlic
A pinch of ground cloves
A pinch of ground allspice
⅛ teaspoon cayenne

- Put all the ingredients in any blender. Blend well until smooth and creamy.

- Pour into a small saucepan. Bring to a boil and simmer for 15 minutes. Serve.

Gluten-free	Dairy-free	Egg-free	Meat-free	Tree Nut–free	Vegan	Diabetic-friendly	Candida-friendly	High-protein	10 minutes or less
●	●	●	●	●	●	●	●		

PALEO SOUR CREAM

Rich, creamy, and dairy-free, this coconut sour cream is free of the chemicals and stabilizers you'll find in commercial brands and is an ideal topping for breakfasts (and lunches and dinners!). This tastes fantastic on omelets (page 199), Wild Salmon Cakes (page 233), and Sweet Potato Latkes (page 123). It's similar to Coconut Cream Topping (page 249), except it's a bit sour. Store in the refrigerator for up to 3 days.

YIELD: ⅔ cup

1 can thick full-fat unsweetened coconut milk (page 13)
1½ tablespoons lemon juice
½ tablespoon apple cider vinegar
⅛ heaping teaspoon unprocessed salt

- Chill the coconut milk in the can overnight, or for 3 to 4 hours, until it thickens into a lovely cream. (Better yet, keep a can in the fridge at all times!)

- Flip the can upside down, open it, and pour off the thin liquid to use in something else. Scrape out the thick cream. Add the lemon juice, vinegar, and salt.

- Whisk until smooth and serve. (If you want it perfectly lump free, process briefly with a mini-blender, immersion blender, or mixer.)

Gluten-free	Dairy-free	Egg-free	Meat-free	Tree Nut–free	Vegan	Diabetic-friendly	Candida-friendly	High-protein	10 minutes or less
●	●	●	●	●	●	●	●		●

PARMESAN CHEESE SAUCE

Coconut butter and nutritional yeast combine for a zesty Italian flavor. This cheesy sauce is dairy-free and so easy to make—just blend and serve. For best results, have all ingredients at room temperature. It tastes amazing on Italian Baked Eggs (page 204) or Open-Faced Focaccia with Sausage (page 179). Freeze leftover sauce in a BPA-free container. Or freeze in an ice cube tray overnight, then store cubes in a freezer bag for up to 3 months, so you can pull out a cube at a time. Or store in the refrigerator for 3 days.

YIELD: 1 cup • **EQUIPMENT:** Small blender, immersion blender with cup, or food processor

½ cup thick full-fat unsweetened coconut milk (page 13)
3 tablespoons nutritional yeast
3 tablespoons lemon juice
1 small clove garlic, crushed or diced (optional)
½ teaspoon unprocessed salt
Black pepper
3 tablespoons (42 grams) Coconut Butter (page 33)
1 tablespoon coconut oil

• Combine the coconut milk, nutritional yeast, lemon juice, garlic (if using), salt, and pepper. Blend well until creamy. Add the coconut butter and coconut oil last and process until smooth. Pour into a serving pitcher. Chill to thicken.

Gluten-free	Dairy-free	Egg-free	Meat-free	Tree Nut–free	Vegan	Diabetic-friendly	Candida-friendly	High-protein	10 minutes or less
●	●	●	●	●	●	●	●		●

SPICY CHEESE SAUCE

You may have noticed that I suggest using this cheese sauce in a lot of finished dishes. That's because the rich, mellow flavor of cheese is so compatible with many savory recipes in this book. Coconut butter, nutritional yeast, and lemon juice provide a subtle cheese taste that's completely vegan and dairy-free. It's so easy to blend, and you can keep it on hand in the freezer. For best results, have all ingredients at room temperature. Try it on Sweet Potato Tots (page 185), Beef Fajitas (page 228), or Personal Pizza for One (page 180) and Open-Faced Focaccia with Sausage (page 179). Freeze leftover sauce in a BPA-free container. Or freeze in an ice cube tray overnight, then put cubes in a freezer bag for up to 3 months, so you can pull out a cube at a time. Or store in the refrigerator for 3 days.

YIELD: 1 cup sauce • **EQUIPMENT:** Any small blender, immersion blender with cup, or food processor

½ cup thick full-fat, unsweetened coconut milk (page 13)
2 tablespoons nutritional yeast
2 tablespoons lemon juice
1 small clove garlic, crushed or diced
½ teaspoon unprocessed salt
Black pepper
½ teaspoon ground mustard
½ teaspoon chili powder
Optional for yellow color: ½ medium grated carrot
3 tablespoons (42 grams) Coconut Butter (page 33)
1 tablespoon coconut oil

- In any small blender, immersion blender with a cup, or food processor, add coconut milk, nutritional yeast, lemon juice, garlic, salt, pepper, mustard, chili powder, and carrot, if using. Blend well until it's a creamy texture. Add the coconut butter and coconut oil last and process until smooth. Pour into a serving pitcher. Chill to thicken.

Gluten-free	Dairy-free	Egg-free	Meat-free	Tree Nut–free	Vegan	Diabetic-friendly	Candida-friendly	High-protein	10 minutes or less
●	●	●	●	●	●	●	●		●

METRIC CONVERSIONS

The recipes in this book have not been tested with metric measurements, so some variations might occur.

Remember that the weight of dry ingredients varies according to the volume or density factor: 1 cup of flour weighs far less than 1 cup of sugar, and 1 tablespoon doesn't necessarily hold 3 teaspoons.

General Formula for Metric Conversion

Ounces to grams	Multiply ounces by 28.35
Grams to ounces	Multiply grams by 0.035
Pounds to grams	Multiply pounds by 453.5
Pounds to kilograms	Multiply pounds by 0.45
Cups to liters	Multiply cups by 0.24
Fahrenheit to Celsius	Subtract 32 from Fahrenheit temperature, multiply by 5, divide by 9
Celsius to Fahrenheit	Multiply Celsius temperature by 9, divide by 5, add 32

Volume (Liquid) Measurements

1 teaspoon = ⅙ fluid ounce = 5 milliliters
1 tablespoon = ½ fluid ounce = 15 milliliters
2 tablespoons = 1 fluid ounce = 30 milliliters
¼ cup = 2 fluid ounces = 60 milliliters
⅓ cup = 2⅔ fluid ounces = 79 milliliters
½ cup = 4 fluid ounces = 118 milliliters
1 cup or ½ pint = 8 fluid ounces = 250 milliliters
2 cups or 1 pint = 16 fluid ounces = 500 milliliters
4 cups or 1 quart = 32 fluid ounces = 1,000 milliliters
1 gallon = 4 liters

Volume (Dry) Measurements

¼ teaspoon = 1 milliliter	½ cup = 118 milliliters
½ teaspoon = 2 milliliters	⅔ cup = 158 milliliters
¾ teaspoon = 4 milliliters	¾ cup = 177 milliliters
1 teaspoon = 5 milliliters	1 cup = 225 milliliters
1 tablespoon = 15 milliliters	4 cups or 1 quart = 1 liter
¼ cup = 59 milliliters	½ gallon = 2 liters
⅓ cup = 79 milliliters	1 gallon = 4 liters

Weight (Mass) Measurements

1 ounce = 30 grams
2 ounces = 55 grams
3 ounces = 85 grams
4 ounces = ¼ pound = 125 grams
8 ounces = ½ pound = 240 grams
12 ounces = ¾ pound = 375 grams
16 ounces = 1 pound = 454 grams

Linear Measure

½ inch = 1⅓ cm
1 inch = 2½ cm
6 inches = 15 cm
8 inches = 20 cm
10 inches = 25 cm
12 inches = 30 cm
20 inches = 50 cm

Oven Temperature Equivalents
Fahrenheit (F) and Celsius (C)

100°F = 38°C
200°F = 95°C
250°F = 120°C
300°F = 150°C
350°F = 180°C
400°F = 205°C
450°F = 230°C

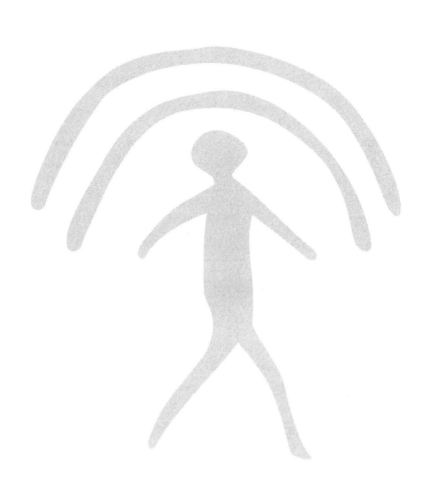

APPENDIX A

CHART OF RECIPES BY DIET

If you're looking for recipes that correspond to a diet, are high in protein, or super-quick, this chart is for you. These Paleo breakfasts are compatible to many alternative diets. All 165 recipes are gluten- and grain-free; 164 are dairy-free. There are 79 egg-free recipes, 101 tree nut–free, 131 meat-free, and 57 vegan recipes. In addition, 162 recipes are diabetic-friendly, and 152 are candida-friendly. There are 79 high-protein recipes. And 68 recipes can be ready to eat in 10 minutes or less.

Besides being Paleo, gluten-free, and celiac-friendly, all these recipes are free of corn, potatoes, peanuts, and soy. If you choose zero-carb sweeteners such as Just Like Sugar, PureLo, or Swerve (page 18), then all recipes

are both diabetic- and candida-friendly. If this is you or someone in your family, I recommend steering completely clear of honey due to its high sugar content. All but one smoothie recipe are dairy-free. Vegan recipes contain no dairy, eggs, meat, honey, or bee pollen. Tree nuts are defined as almonds, walnuts, pecans, cashews, macadamias, hazelnuts, Brazil nuts, and other similar nuts. Note that coconut is not considered a tree nut, nor are seeds such as flaxseeds, hemp seeds, sesame seeds, and pumpkin seeds. If an ingredient is optional, meaning it can be skipped and is not essential to the dish, the recipe is labeled as if it does not contain it.

———

continues

1. Breakfast Staples	Page	Gluten-free	Dairy-free	Egg-free	Meat-free	Tree Nut–free	Vegan	Diabetic-friendly	Candida-friendly	High-protein	10 minutes or less
Coconut Butter	33	•	•	•	•	•	•	•	•		•
Homemade Coconut Milk	35	•	•	•	•	•	•	•	•		•
High-Protein Coconut Milk	35	•	•	•	•	•	•	•	•	•	•
Homemade Nut Milk	36	•	•	•	•		•	•	•		•
High-Protein Nut Milk	37	•	•	•			•	•	•	•	•
Flavored Coconut and Nut Milk	37	•	•	•			•	•	•		•
Homemade Nut Butter	38	•	•	•	•		•	•	•	•	•
Chocolate Nut Butter	39	•	•	•	•		•			•	•
Soaking and Crisping Nuts	40	•	•	•	•		•	•	•	•	
Homemade Bacon Bits	42					•		•		•	
Paleo Cream Cheese	43	•	•	•	•	•	•	•	•		•
Herbed Cream Cheese	43	•	•	•	•	•	•	•	•		•
Paleo Feta Cheese	44	•	•	•	•	•	•	•	•		
Paleo Butter	45	•	•	•	•	•	•	•	•		•
Paleo Omega-3 Butter	45	•	•	•	•	•	•	•	•		•
Perfect Coconut Pie Crust	46	•	•		•	•	•	•			
Homemade Bone Broth	47	•	•	•		•		•		•	
Fermented Veggies	48	•	•	•	•	•	•	•	•		

2. Savory Breads	Page	Gluten-free	Dairy-free	Egg-free	Meat-free	Tree Nut–free	Vegan	Diabetic-friendly	Candida-friendly	High-protein	10 minutes or less
Almond Sandwich Bread	53	•	•		•			•	•	•	
Fluffy Almond Butter Bread	54	•	•		•			•	•	•	
Fluffy White Bread	55	•	•		•	•		•	•		
Cinnamon Swirl Bread	56	•	•		•	•		•	•		
Black Russian Superfood Chocolate Manna Bread	57	•	•		•					•	
Old-World Seed Bread	59	•	•		•			•		•	

2. Savory Breads	Page	Gluten-free	Dairy-free	Egg-free	Meat-free	Tree Nut–free	Vegan	Diabetic-friendly	Candida-friendly	High-protein	10 minutes or less
Pumpernickel Rye Bread	61	●	●		●			●	●	●	
Rosemary Olive Bread	63	●	●		●			●	●	●	
Sour Cream Onion Dill Bread	65	●	●		●			●	●	●	
English Muffins	67	●	●		●	●		●	●		
Baking Powder Biscuits	68	●	●		●			●	●	●	
Chili Cheese Biscuits	69	●	●		●			●	●		
Sweet Potato Rosemary Biscuits	70	●	●		●			●	●		
Bacon Chili Cornbread	71	●	●					●	●		
Classic Cornbread or Corn Muffins	72	●	●		●			●	●		
Chia Corn Tortillas	73	●	●		●	●		●	●		
Plantain Tortillas	75	●	●	●	●	●	●	●	●		
Easy Burrito Wraps	76	●	●		●	●		●	●		
Focaccia Flat Bread, Egg-Free	77	●	●		●		●	●	●		
Garlic Naan	78	●	●		●			●	●		

3. Instant Smoothies, Beverages, and Parfaits	Page	Gluten-free	Dairy-free	Egg-free	Meat-free	Tree Nut–free	Vegan	Diabetic-friendly	Candida-friendly	High-protein	10 minutes or less
Blueberry Orange Smoothie	80	●	●	●	●	●	●	●	●	●	●
Berry Grapefruit Smoothie with Greens	82	●	●	●	●	●	●	●	●	●	●
Chocolate Almond Pick-Me-Up	83	●	●	●	●					●	●
Cran-Apple Spice Smoothie	84	●	●	●	●	●	●	●	●	●	●
High-Protein Kefir Berry Smoothie	85	●		●	●			●		●	●
Papaya Berry Smoothie	86	●	●	●	●	●	●	●	●	●	●
Peaches and Greens Smoothie	87	●	●	●	●	●	●	●	●	●	●
Strawberry Beet Smoothie	88	●	●	●	●	●	●	●	●	●	●
Sunrise Green Smoothie	89	●	●	●	●		●	●	●	●	●

3. Instant Smoothies, Beverages, and Parfaits	Page	Gluten-free	Dairy-free	Egg-free	Meat-free	Tree Nut-free	Vegan	Diabetic-friendly	Candida-friendly	High-protein	10 minutes or less
Fruit with Coconut Cream Topping	90	●	●	●	●	●	●	●	●		●
Blue Mousse	91	●	●	●	●	●	●	●	●		●
Raspberry Cheesecake Parfait	92	●	●	●	●		●	●	●		●
Chia Tapioca Fruit Parfait	93	●	●	●	●	●	●	●	●		●
Lemon Berry Parfait	94	●	●	●	●		●	●	●		●
Pumpkin Banana Nut Parfait	95	●	●	●	●		●	●	●		●
Blueberry Hemp Parfait	96	●	●	●	●	●	●	●	●	●	●
Vanilla Cream Parfait with Strawberries and Pumpkin Seeds	97	●	●	●	●		●	●			
Cappuccino	98	●	●	●	●	●	●	●	●		●
Caffè Latte	98	●	●	●	●	●	●	●	●		●
Mochaccino	98	●	●	●	●	●	●	●	●		●
Chai Tea	99	●	●	●	●	●	●	●	●		●

4. Grain Free Cereals	Page	Gluten-free	Dairy-free	Egg-free	Meat-free	Tree Nut-free	Vegan	Diabetic-friendly	Candida-friendly	High-protein	10 minutes or less
Apple Cinnamon Granola	103	●	●	●	●		●	●	●		
Cocoa-Nutty Granola	104	●	●	●	●						
High-Protein Chia Crunch Granola	105	●	●	●	●					●	
Cream of Hemp with Apple and Cinnamon	106	●	●	●	●	●	●	●	●	●	●
Coconut Flax Cereal with Berries	107	●	●	●	●		●	●	●		●
Flax Oatmeal with Banana	108	●	●	●	●		●	●			●
Coconut Panna Cotta with Honey and Walnuts	109	●	●	●	●		●	●	●		
Coconut Panna Cotta with Berries and Nuts	109	●	●	●	●		●	●	●		
Cauliflower Rice Pudding	110	●	●	●	●		●	●	●		
Kasha with Bacon and Mushrooms	111	●	●	●		●		●			

5. Griddle Goodies	Page	Gluten-free	Dairy-free	Egg-free	Meat-free	Tree Nut–free	Vegan	Diabetic-friendly	Candida-friendly	High-protein	10 minutes or less
Banana Nut Pancakes with Cardamom	115	•	•		•			•	•		
Blueberry Pancakes	117	•	•		•			•	•		
Traditional Plantain Pancakes	119	•	•		•			•	•		
Zucchini Pancakes	121	•	•		•			•	•		
Sweet Potato Latkes	123	•	•		•	•		•	•		
Sweet Potato Pancakes	124	•	•		•			•	•		
Chocolate Brownie Superfood Waffles	125	•	•		•			•	•		
Pecan Waffles	127	•	•		•			•	•	•	
Sour Cream Waffles	128	•	•		•	•		•	•		
Squash Bacon Waffles with Pecans	129	•	•					•	•	•	
Cinnamon Swirl French Toast	131	•	•		•	•		•	•		•
Baked French Toast	132	•	•		•	•		•	•		
Perfect Paleo Crepes	133	•	•		•	•		•	•	•	•
Crepes Suzette	134	•	•		•	•		•	•	•	
Apple Fritters	135	•	•		•			•	•		

6. Sweet Quick Breads and Muffins	Page	Gluten-free	Dairy-free	Egg-free	Meat-free	Tree Nut–free	Vegan	Diabetic-friendly	Candida-friendly	High-protein	10 minutes or less
Banana Bread	139	•	•		•			•	•		
Chocolate Pumpkin Bread	140	•	•		•			•	•		
Cranberry Orange Cardamom Bread	141	•	•		•			•	•		
Lemon Bread	142	•	•		•			•	•		
Lemon Ginger Bread with Basil	142	•	•		•			•	•		
Lemon Poppyseed Bread	142	•	•		•			•	•		
Old-World Sweet Potato Bread with Pecans	143	•	•		•			•	•		
Zucchini Bread	144	•	•		•			•	•		

6. Sweet Quick Breads and Muffins	Page	Gluten-free	Dairy-free	Egg-free	Meat-free	Tree Nut–free	Vegan	Diabetic-friendly	Candida-friendly	High-protein	10 minutes or less
Chocolate Zucchini Bread	144	•	•		•			•	•		
Apple Spice Muffins, Egg-Free	145	•	•	•	•		•	•	•		
Blueberry Lemon Muffins	147	•	•		•			•	•		
Cranberry Pecan Muffins	148	•	•		•			•	•		
Lemon Chia Seed Muffins, Egg-Free	149	•	•	•	•		•	•	•		
Pumpkin Muffins with Streusel Topping	150	•	•		•			•	•		
Cinnamon Apple Sour Cream Coffeecake Muffins	152	•	•		•			•	•		

7. Bars, Crumbles, and Other Sweets	Page	Gluten-free	Dairy-free	Egg-free	Meat-free	Tree Nut–free	Vegan	Diabetic-friendly	Candida-friendly	High-protein	10 minutes or less
Big Breakfast Cookies	157	•	•		•			•	•	•	
Blueberry Crumble Bars	158	•	•	•	•		•	•	•	•	
Caramel Chocolate Superfood Bars	160	•	•		•			•		•	
Apple Bread Pudding	162		•		•	•		•			
Apple Berry Crisp	163	•	•	•	•		•	•	•		
Pear Ginger Crisp with Berries	164	•	•	•	•		•	•	•		
Peach Shortbread Crumble	165	•	•		•			•	•		
Blueberry Cobbler in a Cup	166	•	•		•			•	•		
Strawberry Rhubarb Cobbler in a Cup	166	•	•		•			•	•		
Sweet Potato Popovers	167	•	•		•	•		•	•		

8. My Dad's Favorite Hearty Breakfasts	Page	Gluten-free	Dairy-free	Egg-free	Meat-free	Tree Nut–free	Vegan	Diabetic-friendly	Candida-friendly	High-protein	10 minutes or less
Sweet Potato Hash with Turkey Apple Sausage	170	•	•			•		•		•	
Bacon Cauliflower Hash with Eggs	171	•	•			•		•	•	•	

8. My Dad's Favorite Hearty Breakfasts	Page	Gluten-free	Dairy-free	Egg-free	Meat-free	Tree Nut–free	Vegan	Diabetic-friendly	Candida-friendly	High-protein	10 minutes or less
Design Your Own Hash Browns	173	●	●			●		●	●	●	
Wild Salmon Cauliflower Hash	174	●	●			●		●	●	●	
Biscuits and Gravy	176	●	●					●	●	●	
Breakfast Burritos	177	●	●			●		●	●	●	
Breakfast Tacos	178	●	●			●		●	●	●	
Open-Faced Focaccia with Sausage	179	●	●	●				●	●	●	
Personal Pizza for One	180	●	●					●	●	●	
Quesadillas	181	●	●			●		●	●	●	
Southwest Vegetable Fritters	182	●	●		●	●		●	●		
Spicy Southwest Breakfast Pockets	183	●	●					●	●	●	
Sweet Potato Tots	185	●	●	●	●	●	●	●			
Cauliflower Tater Tots	185	●	●	●	●	●	●	●			
Tamale Pie	186	●	●					●	●	●	
Egg Foo Yong	188	●	●		●	●		●	●	●	●
Cauliflower Fried Rice	189	●	●		●	●		●	●		●
Egg Drop Soup	191	●	●		●	●		●	●	●	●
Pho Ga, Vietnamese Chicken Soup	192	●	●	●		●		●	●	●	●
Zoodle Soup	193	●	●	●	●	●	●	●	●	●	●

9. The Egg Always Comes First	Page	Gluten-free	Dairy-free	Egg-free	Meat-free	Tree Nut–free	Vegan	Diabetic-friendly	Candida-friendly	High-protein	10 minutes or less
Asparagus Frittata with Herbs and Cream Cheese	197	●	●		●	●		●	●	●	
Bacon-Wrapped Eggs	198	●	●			●		●		●	
Classic Omelet with Eighteen Variations	199	●	●			●		●	●	●	●
Baked Eggs in Portobello Mushroom with Bacon	202	●	●			●		●		●	

10. Meats and Other Wild Breakfasts	Page	Gluten-free	Dairy-free	Egg-free	Meat-free	Tree Nut–free	Vegan	Diabetic-friendly	Candida-friendly	High-protein	10 minutes or less
Beef Fajitas with Spicy Cheese Sauce	228	•	•	•		•		•	•	•	•
Chicken Adobo on Tortillas	229	•	•	•		•		•	•	•	•
Chicken Livers with Bacon on Toast	230	•	•	•		•		•	•	•	•
Easy Liver Pâté	231	•	•	•		•		•	•	•	
Sautéed Kidney with Onions and Lemon	232	•	•	•		•		•	•	•	
Wild Salmon Cakes with Sour Cream	233	•	•					•	•	•	
Wild Salmon with Garlicky Greens	234	•	•	•		•		•	•	•	

Sausage:	Page	Gluten-free	Dairy-free	Egg-free	Meat-free	Tree Nut–free	Vegan	Diabetic-friendly	Candida-friendly	High-protein	10 minutes or less
Homemade Breakfast Sausage	235	•	•	•		•		•	•	•	
Green Chile Lamb Sausage	236	•	•	•		•		•	•	•	
Spicy Chorizo	237	•	•	•		•		•	•	•	
Turkey Sausage with Apple and Sage	238	•	•	•		•		•	•	•	
Zesty Italian Sausage	239	•	•	•		•		•		•	

11. Sauces, Toppings, and Jams	Page	Gluten-free	Dairy-free	Egg-free	Meat-free	Tree Nut–free	Vegan	Diabetic-friendly	Candida-friendly	High-protein	10 minutes or less
Berrylicious Sauce	243	•	•	•	•	•	•	•	•		•
Blackberry Sauce	243	•	•	•	•	•	•	•	•		•
Blueberry Chia Jam	244	•	•	•	•	•	•	•	•		•
Orange Marmalade	245	•	•	•	•	•	•	•	•		
Maple Flavor Syrup	246	•	•	•	•	•	•	•	•		•
Maple Pecan Syrup	246	•	•	•	•		•	•	•		•
Orange Maple Syrup	246	•	•	•	•	•	•	•	•		•
Ginger Cardamom Syrup	247	•	•	•	•	•	•	•	•		•
Hot Caramel Sauce	248	•		•	•	•	•	•	•		•
Coconut Cream Topping	249	•	•	•	•	•	•	•	•		•

11. Sauces, Toppings, and Jams	Page	Gluten-free	Dairy-free	Egg-free	Meat-free	Tree Nut–free	Vegan	Diabetic-friendly	Candida-friendly	High-protein	10 minutes or less
Chipotle Butter	250	●	●	●	●	●					●
Orange Honey Butter	251	●	●	●	●	●					●
Avocado Pesto	252	●	●	●	●	●	●	●	●		●
Cilantro Pesto	253	●	●	●	●	●	●	●	●		●
Hollandaise Sauce	254	●	●	●	●	●	●	●	●		●
Homemade Ketchup	255	●	●	●	●	●	●	●	●		
Paleo Sour Cream	256	●	●	●	●	●	●	●	●		●
Parmesan Cheese Sauce	257	●	●	●	●	●	●	●	●		●
Spicy Cheese Sauce	258	●	●	●	●	●	●	●	●		●

APPENDIX B

RESOURCES—BUYING GUIDE

Depending on where you live, you may be able to get many of these ingredients at your local health food store. You can also buy online (often in bulk—more economical). Here are some of my go-to resources for ingredients used in these recipes.

INGREDIENTS:	
Açaí Berries, Sambazon Smoothie Packs, unsweetened	amazon.com
Agar powder	Frontier brand at amazon.com
Almond meal	bobsredmill.com, vitacost.com
Apple cider vinegar	bragg.com, vitacost.com
Arrowroot flour	bobsredmill.com, vitacost.com
Baking soda	any grocery
Bee pollen	iherb.com, vitacost.com
Buckwheat	bobsredmill.com, vitacost.com
Cacao powder, cacao nibs	vitacost.com, navitasnaturals.com, sunfood.com
Carob powder	bobsredmill.com, vitacost.com
Chia seeds, both black and white	nutiva.com, vitacost.com
Chicory root granules, roasted	frontiercoop.com, amazon.com
Chlorella powder	sunfood.com, mountainroseherbs.com, vitacost.com
ChlorOxygen	luckyvitamin.com, vitacost.com
Coconut aminos	iherb.com, vitacost.com
Coconut butter	artisanafoods.com, vitacost.com
Coconut flour	bobsredmill.com, vitacost.com
Coconut milk, canned	edwardandsons.com, naturalvalue.com, vitacost.com

 continues

INGREDIENTS:	
Coconut oil	tropicaltraditions.com, vitacost.com, nutiva.com
Coconut water, unsweetened	any grocery
Coconut, shredded unsweetened full-fat	vitacost.com, tropicaltraditions.com
Mount Hagen Organic Coffee Café Decaffeinated	vitacost.com, amazon.com
Crystals, Vitamin C	iherb.com, vitacost.com
Dandelion root granules, roasted	Frontier brand at amazon.com
Eggs, pastured organic	Farm direct or organic pasture-raised
Flax seeds, flax meal, and flax oil	bobsredmill.com, vitacost.com
Goat kefir	Any healthy grocery
Goji berries	navitasnaturals.com, vitacost.com
Hemp nuts	nutiva.com, vitacost.com
Holy basil or Tulsi tea in bulk	swansonvitamins.com, iherb.com, starwest-botanicals.com, oregonswildharvest.com
Honey, raw local	honeylocator.com, swansonvitamins.com, vitacost.com
Just Like Sugar Brown	vitacost.com, justlikesugar.com
Just Like Sugar Table Top	vitacost.com, justlikesugar.com
Maca powder	navitasnaturals.com, vitacost.com
Maple flavor	baktoflavors.com
Meats and poultry, grass-fed, and wild fish	eatwild.com
Nutritional yeast	bragg.com, bobsredmill.com, vitacost.com
Nuts and seeds	sunorganicfarm.com, tierrafarm.com, rawnutsandseeds.com, wildernessfamilynaturals.com
Onion flakes	wildernessfamilynaturals.com, frontier.com
Protein powder—100 percent egg whites	nowfoods.com
Protein powder-Bluebonnet Whey Protein Isolate Original Unsweetened	iherb.com
PureLo Lo Han Sweetener	swansonvitamins.com, amazon.com
Red palm oil	tropicaltraditions.com, nutiva.com
Salt, unprocessed	swansonvitamins.com, vitacost.com
Seaweed, hiziki, and wakame	edenfoods.com, vitacost.com
Sweeteners:	swervesweetener.com
Swerve Sweetener	mountainroseherbs.com
Vitamin-C Crystals	iherb.com, vitacost.com

SUPPLIES:	
Food processor	cuisinart.com, kitchenaid.com
Glass bread pan	World Kitchen-Pyrex/Corelle 1 ½ Qt Pyrex Loaf Dish at amazon.com
Hand-held grinder	Krups 203 Electric Coffee and Spice Grinder
High-speed blender	blendtec.com, vitamix.com
Immersion blender with cup	Cuisinart SmartStick Handblender at cuisinart.com, amazon.com
Mason jars	amazon.com
Milk frother for cappuccino	Aerolatte at amazon.com
Nut milk bag	amazon.com
Spiral Vegetable Slicer	Saladacco Spiral Slicer, the Paderno World Cuisine Tri-Blade Plastic Spiral Vegetable Slicer, or any stainless steel mandoline slicer at Amazon

FOR MORE INFORMATION:

Balanced Bites—balancedbites.com

A highly informative blog by Diane Sanfilippo, talented author of *Practical Paleo*. Her 21-Day Sugar Detox program is the best I've seen.

Chris Kresser—chriskresser.com

A licensed acupuncturist, practitioner of integrative medicine, and author of *Beyond Paleo*, Chris's blog contains a wealth of reliable information about health and diet.

Everyday Paleo—everydaypaleo.com

Sarah Fragoso is a fitness trainer, mother, and author of several excellent books on the Paleo diet. Her blog contains recipes and articles on fitness.

Good Morning Paleo—goodmorningpaleo.com

This is my website for this book. It contains greater in-depth information about Paleo breakfasts, free recipes, and a sortable chart by diet.

The Healthy GF Life—thehealthygflife.com

Tammy Credicott is the author of *Paleo Indulgences*, *The Healthy Gluten Free Life*, and *Make Ahead Paleo*. Her blog The Healthy GF Life is full of recipes and ideas for gluten-free Paleo families.

Jane's Healthy Kitchen—janeshealthykitchen.com

This is my website for health tips and luscious original recipes of all types. This is where I post discoveries of exciting new ways to prepare food for alternative diets and everybody.

Mark's Daily Apple—marksdailyapple.com

Health and fitness expert Mark Sisson is the bestselling author of *The Primal Blueprint* and a leading voice in the Evolutionary Health Movement. His blog is a valuable resource and forum. Mark's mission is to empower people to take responsibility for their health and well-being.

Paleo Desserts—paleodesserts.com

This website is for my book *Paleo Desserts*. It contains articles and in-depth information about how to create healthy sweets, free recipes, and support for people kicking the sugar habit without deprivation.

The Paleo Diet—thepaleodiet.com

Dr. Loren Cordain, Ph.D., is the world's leading expert on Paleolithic diets and founder of the Paleo movement. His book *The Paleo Diet* led the way for widespread interest in the ancestral diet. His blog contains information about the Paleo diet for health and research that supports it.

Paleo Magazine—paleomagonline.com

Paleo Magazine was founded by Cain Credicott in 2011. It is a rich resource and blog about the Paleo diet with a wide range of recipes, fitness tips, and lifestyle topics.

Perfect Health Diet—perfecthealthdiet.com

Paul Jaminet, Ph.D, a former Harvard astrophysicist, and his wife Shou-Ching, a molecular biologist, are scientists with a long-standing interest in health. They are co-authors of *The Perfect Health Diet: Regain Health and Lose Weight by Eating the Way You Were Meant to Eat*. Their blog is a wealth of information on diet, recipes, and other resources.

Robb Wolf—robbwolf.com

A former research biochemist, Robb Wolf wrote the bestselling book *The Paleo Solution*. A student of Dr. Loren Cordain, author of *The Paleo Diet*, Robb offers vital information via his iTunes podcasts, books, and seminars.

Weston Price Foundation—westonaprice.org

A nonprofit organization founded to disseminate the research of Dr. Weston Price, nutrition pioneer. Dr. Price's work demonstrated that humans achieve perfect physical health generation after generation only when they consume nutrient-dense whole foods and animal fats. This website is a rich source of research and practical solutions in diet and health.

ACKNOWLEDGMENTS

*"I've failed over and over and over again
in my life, and that is why I succeed."*
—Michael Jordan

Thanks most of all to you, my readers and subscribers at JanesHealthyKitchen.com and PaleoDesserts.com, for your encouragement, e-mails, and requests.

A bow of gratitude to Qigong and Yoga Master Zhenzan Dao of mogadao.com, who inspired this book from the start, gifting it with his intelligence, wit, and sensitivity. He personally tasted almost every recipe with the goal of inventing nutrient-dense meals of authentic Paleo ingredients, in order to balance and cultivate qi while also pleasing the senses. You'll find his enthusiasm, patience, and candid feedback on every page, although his words are silent. I'll tell you a secret—his favorite recipe is Pumpernickel Bread. Oh, and he panned quite a few recipes that didn't make it into the book, such as waterlogged egg-free quiche and Paleo baguettes that caused a Pyrex pan to explode all over my kitchen.

To my many taste-testers, I offer thundering applause, especially Tyler White, Johana Moore, Sunny Smyth, Nikesha Breeze, Lissa Reidel, and Orlando Leibovitz, who put away countless breakfasts, giving their honest comments and encouragement.

Thank you to Fred Brown for his guidance, helping me to create the book concept and contents with integrity and spirit.

Infinite appreciation goes to my executive editor, Renee Sedliar, for her original idea, her perseverance, and for making my writing so much better than it is. Thank you to Isabelle Bleeker for her contribution and guidance. To my project editor, Carolyn Sobczak, gratitude for her careful work and for putting up with my constant changes, and also to my copy editor, Martha Whitt—I gave her a big job! Thanks to designers Trish Wilkinson, Alex Camlin, and photographer Lloyd Lemmermann. And a kiss to my sister, Ann, for her wise words.

INDEX